GARLAND STUDIES ON
THE ELDERLY IN AMERICA

edited by
STUART BRUCHEY
UNIVERSITY OF MAINE

A GARLAND SERIES

RACIAL DIFFERENCES IN LIFE EXPECTANCY AMONG ELDERLY AFRICAN AMERICANS AND WHITES

The Surprising Truth about Comparisons

LAURA B. SHRESTHA

GARLAND PUBLISHING, INC.
NEW YORK & LONDON / 1997

Copyright © 1997 Laura B. Shrestha
All rights reserved

Library of Congress Cataloging-in-Publication Data

Shrestha, Laura B.
  Racial differences in life expectancy among elderly African Americans and whites : the surprising truth about comparisons / Laura B. Shrestha.
    p.   cm. — (Garland studies on the elderly in America)
  Includes bibliographical references and index.
  ISBN 0-8153-2764-1 (alk. paper)
  1. Afro-American aged—Mortality. 2. Aged—United States—Mortality. 3. Life expectancy—United States. I. Title. II. Series.
HB1323.B5S55 1997
304.6'45'08996073—dc21   96-30016

Printed on acid-free, 250-year-life paper
Manufactured in the United States of America

r 304.645 S561r 1997
Shrestha, Laura B.
Racial differences in life
expectancy among elderly

Dedication

This book is dedicated to my family. Thank you to my mother, Helen L. Arthur, for your persistent encouragement of higher education and for your undying pride in your family. Gratitude to my husband TJ and daughters Lena (age 8) and June (age 5) Shrestha for your forbearance and sympathetic support during the writing of this book.

Contents

	List of tables, illustration, and figures	ix
	Preface	xi
	Acknowledgments	xiii
I.	Overview	3
	Some ambiguities in the U.S. Data	6
	A Brief Description of Future Chapters	10
II.	Quality of Census Data on the Older Population	13
	Background	13
	General Methods for Evaluating Census Coverage and Content Errors	18
	Evaluation of the 1970 Census	20
	Evaluation of the 1980 Census	39
	Evaluation of the 1990 Census	48
	Age Heaping and Racial Misclassification	53
III.	Evaluation of Death Registration and Immigration Statistics	57
	Death Registration Data	57
	The Immigration Statistics	70
IV.	Adjustments to the Data Sources	73
	Adjustments to the 1970 Census	76
	Adjustments to the 1980 Census	83
	Adjustments to the 1990 Census	88
	The Vital Registration System	95
	Net Immigration Statistics	97

V.	Simulated Effects of Coverage and Reporting Errors	105
	An Intercensal Methodology to Evaluate Quality of Old-Age Data	106
	How Age Overstatement Affects the Ratios, based on Simulation Results	107
	Deriving Estimates of "True" 1980 and 1990 Population Age Distributions and Intercensal Deaths	111
VI.	U.S. Results: Errors in the Ratios and their Effects on Life Expectancy	131
	Results for Whites	136
	Results for Blacks	
	Summary	
VII.	Bibliography	155
VIII.	Author Index	167
IX.	Content Index	169

List of Tables, Illustrations or Figures

Tables

1.1	Population aged 65+, United States	5
1.2	Persons aged 100+ among those aged 65+	7
2.1	Characteristic allocation in censuses	16
2.2	Underenumeration in 1970 census	23-24
2.3	Undercount of black females-1970 census	26
2.4	Gross missed rates in 1970 census	29
2.5	Illustrative table to estimate reporting accuracy	30
2.6	Indices of age reporting errors in 1970 census	32-33
2.7	Consistency between CPS and census, 1970	36-37
2.8	Underenumeration in 1980 census	42-43
2.9	Undercount in 1980 by different methodologies	46-47
2.10	Undercount in 1990 census	
2.11	Consistency between CPS and census, 1990	52
3.1	Age of decedent, 1986 NMFS	59
3.2	Race of decedent, 1986 NMFS	59
3.3	Comparability of age of decedent, two sources	60
3.4	Agreement between death certificate and Medicare	62
3.5	Age agreement-census & matched death certificate	66-67
3.6	Age agreement, New Jersey	68-69
4.1	Centenarian estimates	79-80
4.2	US population size, 1970	82
4.3	Racial identification in the 1980 census	84
4.4	US population size, 1980	86
4.5	US population size, 1990	89
4.6	Deaths in parallelogram	96
4.7	Components of population change, 1970 to 1980	98-100
5.1	Patterns of age misreporting, base on simulations	108
5.2	Estimates of "true" population and deaths	117-119
5.3	Simulations with introduced coverage error	121-122
5.4	Simulations with patterns of age misreporting	125-127
6.1	Results, ratios of observed to expected population	135
6.2	Myers' preference index, white males, 1970-1980	138
6.3	Myers' preference index, black males, 1970-1980	147

Figures

5.1	Simulated pattern - errors in two censuses	109
5.2	Simulated pattern - errors in censuses and deaths	110
5.3	Simulated pattern - differing error	111
6.1	Results: whites, by sex, 1970-1980	136
6.2	Results: whites, by sex, 1980-1990	143
6.3	Results: blacks, by sex, 1970-1980	144
6.4	Results: blacks, by sex, 1980-1990	144

Preface

This book is based on a dissertation written while a student in the Population Studies Center of the University of Pennsylvania, under the guidance of Dr. Samuel H. Preston. The catalyst for the research was the recognition that major uncertainties exist about the quality of population and death data for the elderly in the United States as a result of coverage and content errors in the censuses and death registration. Furthermore, different patterns appear to exist for the two major racial groupings in the United States: whites and African-Americans.

Racial differences in life expectancy have long been observed in the United States, wherein African-American life expectancy at various ages is generally lower than that of whites. At the advanced ages, however, a reversal is observed whereby blacks have more years remaining on average than whites. Is the crossover "real", reflecting some type of biological superiority for African Americans at the oldest ages, or is the phenomenon simply attributable to the poor quality of the data on which mortality statistics are calculated?

The book evaluates the consistency of reported data between the two major sources of data for calculation of mortality statistics in the United States: censuses and death registration. The focus is on the older population (aged 60 and above), where mortality trends have the greatest impact on social programs and where data quality is most problematic. Using demographic techniques, age-specific inconsistencies between the sources are evaluated for both whites and African-Americans for two periods: 1970-1980 and 1980-1990.

While the catalyst for this book was to highlight the effect of age misreporting on mortality estimates in the United States, the evaluation clearly reveals serious consequences for any research that is based on official population and vital registration data at advanced ages.

Acknowledgments

I was fortunate to have been introduced and guided in my demographic studies by a cadre of excellent instructors. First and foremost, I would like to acknowledge Dr. Samuel H. Preston, who played many roles, including dissertation adviser, mentor, classroom professor in "demographic methods", and project director of the African American Mortality Project. Much of the credit for the completion of this project is directly the result of Sam's intervention, through selection of the topic, to professional guidance in the use of the methodologies, and to the interpretation of the results.

I would also like to express gratitude to Dr. Irma Elo and Dr. Douglas Ewbank, members of the dissertation committee for this project. The final product was significantly improved by their substantive contributions and through their meticulous attention to detail.

Many other people contributed to this project. Special thanks to Tania Bissell and to Kristi Long of Garland Publishing for their excellent editing skills and for their patience support in helping me to complete the manuscript on a reasonable time schedule.

Racial Differences in Life Expectancy among Elderly African Americans and Whites

I

Overview

The focus of this book is to evaluate and improve estimates of race-, sex-, and age-specific census enumerations and death registration for the elderly United States population over the period 1970 to 1990. Directly calculated estimates at very high ages are known to be untrustworthy due to conspicuous inconsistencies that result from coverage errors in the census enumerations, possible incompleteness of the death registration, and, especially, characteristic (age, race, etc.) misstatement in vital statistics and in censuses. While the magnitude and direction of the errors have been the subjects of much speculation in the professional literature, little research has been conducted to evaluate and improve age data in the primary data sources. Therefore, the central focus in this book will be on evaluation of age misreporting, which preliminary analysis suggests is the dominant contributor to data inconsistencies in the U.S. populations.

Age misreporting refers to the intentional or inadvertent introduction of errors into reported age data. Various sources of error exist. An *interviewed person* may not be able to provide real ages for himself and for other household members due to ignorance of exact age or because of a wish to intentionally distort the truth. For instance, a person currently receiving payments through entitlement programs based on an incorrect age could be expected to continue to report the incorrect age. Shryock and Siegel (1976) further describe a notable tendency to report an age over 100 for persons of very advanced age stemming from a desire to share in the esteem generally accorded extreme old age or from gross ignorance of the true age. Although likely to affect only small numbers because of the self-reporting of characteristics in the U.S. censuses, the *interviewer* may also introduce bias by estimating an individual's age through visible signs of age or through the use of life cycle events, such as marital status, parity, the birth of grandchildren, etc. *Coding and data processing* can also introduce age errors, by incorrect coding on the interview schedule, or when transferring that data to the computer, or when assigning attributes (Ewbank, 1981; Pressat, 1985).

For the elderly population in the United States, "age misreporting" is generally assumed to be dominated by overstatement of age. For example, in analyzing the 1980 registered deaths and enumerated census, Coale and Kisker (1990) found conclusive evidence of age exaggeration at ages over 95 and persuasive evidence thereof for ages 70 through 95. They further note that greater flaws exist for the nonwhite population relative to the white. The U.S. Bureau of the Census (1984a) compared individual records from different sources and found that the inconsistency in age data increases with age, and that age tends to be overstated. In the same study, the authors found that, in 1970, perhaps 2 percent of the total population reported to be 65 or older was actually under 65. The proportion for nonwhite males was 9 percent. In a record linkage study, in which a sample of death records for the extreme aged in Pennsylvania and New Jersey whose deaths occurred in the 1968 to 1972 time period were matched to the 1900 census enumeration, Rosenwaike and Logue (1983) found a high level of age agreement for whites up to age 100. For non-whites, however, the level of age agreement was substantially lower.

Despite evidence of inconsistencies, researchers have generally accepted the uncertainties associated with the distorted age distributions or have used model-based abstractions of the proposed relationship between a variable and age. For instance, in calculating mortality rates, which depend on both the estimated number of deaths and enumerations of the population, demographers have used empirical schedules that stop at an early open-ended age group (e.g. 80+). Beyond that point, the age pattern of mortality is assumed to follow one of several functional forms (Condran, Himes, and Preston, 1991). While such assumptions may have been adequate in the past, the increasing size (Table 1.1) and importance of the U.S. elderly population mandates further research to update our understanding of the levels and age patterns of mortality at the advanced ages.

Aside from demographic considerations, an evaluation of age misreporting in the elderly population is relevant from a policy perspective. Projection of the health and institutionalization needs of the future old-age population will be enhanced by accurate portrayal of the current population. Furthermore, correct estimation of the size and attributes of the expanding geriatric population will further facilitate calculation of funding needs for both government (Social Security, Medicare, etc.) and private (retirement, life insurance, etc.) programs.

Table 1.1

Estimated and Projected Size of the Population Aged 65+ in Absolute Numbers and as a Proportion of the Total Population: United States, Various Years

Year	Total Population (Thousands)	Population Aged 65+ (Thousands)	Population Aged 65+ as a Proportion of Total Population
1900	76,094	3,100	4.1
1930	123,077	6,706	5.4
1960	180,671	16,675	9.2
1980	227,757	25,704	11.3
2000[1]	268,266	34,882	13.0

Sources: (1) U.S. Bureau of the Census. 1960. *Historical statistics of the United States: Colonial Times to 1957*. A Statistical Abstract Supplement. Series A. pp.22-23. (2) U.S. Bureau of the Census. 1987c. *Statistical Abstract of the United States: 1988*. (108th Edition). Table Numbers 13 and 16.

Notes: (1) Projected (middle series). (2) All estimates as of July 1. Includes Armed Forces Abroad.

A further practical reason exists for studying these data inconsistencies. The censuses and vital registration, in their roles as primary data sources, are often used by practitioners who are not well-versed in the inaccuracies present in the old age mortality statistics. The implication is that any study of the elderly population, undertaken without consideration of the inherent inconsistencies in the reporting of age, could reach false conclusions. Research topics that could benefit from an understanding of age misreporting in the aged population are far-reaching, but include: (1) the economic implications of an expanding dependency ratio, (2) an analysis of the prevalence of medical intervention in the very old population, (3) the effect of divorce on future inter-generational transfers between adult children and their (divorced) parents, (4) calculation of actuarial tables, and (5) calculation of mortality schedules.

Because it is expected that the results of this book will bear on specific issues related to data ambiguities, I will begin with a brief discussion of recent concerns which may be related to data inadequacies.

This presentation will include a comparison of the enumerated, improbably large U.S. centenarian population with the centenarian populations of the Netherlands and Sweden, low-mortality countries chosen for their known accuracy of reporting. A second topic will address the so-called U.S. racial mortality crossover. Blacks at the oldest ages in the U.S. have long experienced lower death rates than whites although the reverse is true at younger ages. A lively theoretical debate has ensued in the professional literature, with one side proposing that blacks who have survived the excessive environmental stresses of their younger years may be destined by natural selection to live an especially long life (U.S. Bureau of the Census, 1984a; McCord and Freeman, 1990). The competing camp (Coale and Kisker, 1990; Zelnik, 1969; Preston et al, 1991), however, maintains that age misreporting and other data inaccuracies, particularly for the black population, have seriously biased the death rates at the oldest ages.

SOME AMBIGUITIES IN U.S. DATA

The U.S. Centenarian Population

Official data sources present an unsteady view of the U.S. centenarian population. In the 1970 census, 106,441 persons aged 100 and over were enumerated, but subsequent analysis by Siegel and Passel (1976) indicated that misunderstanding of the census form and processing errors led to a large over-count of centenarians. They estimated that the correct count should have been in the range of 3,000 to 8,000. In the 1980 census, 32,000 centenarians were counted. But ensuing research by the U.S. Bureau of the Census (1987b) suggested that processing errors and respondent error again caused a large overcount. The correct count of centenarians should have been around 15,000. In the 1990 official tabulations, 37,306 individuals are aged 100 and over. The Census Bureau deflated its centenarian estimate to 35,808 in subsequent tabulations to be utilized in its estimates and projections program (Word and Spencer, 1991).

While the exact number of centenarians is unknown, simple calculations suggest that their number is almost certainly overestimated. Referring to Table 1.2, which presents comparative data for the United States in 1980, the Netherlands from 1976-80, and Sweden from 1978-82, we can estimate the proportion of centenarians among those aged 65 and above. This proportion can then be used to compare the U.S. population to other low-mortality populations with accurate data.

Table 1.2

Proportion of Persons Aged 100+ Among Those Aged 65+:
Selected Populations, Various Years (per 1000)

Population	Proportion Aged 100+ Among Persons Aged 65+	
	Males	Females
United States, 1980		
Whites	0.81	1.23
Blacks	2.95	3.61
Netherlands, 1976-80	0.16	0.26
Sweden, 1978-82	0.14	0.31

Sources: adapted from the following: (1) Coale and Kisker, 1990. Defects in data on old-age mortality in the United States: new procedures for calculating mortality schedules and life tables at the highest ages. *Asian and Pacific Population Forum*. 4(1), table 2; (2) U.S. Bureau of the Census, 1987b. Current Population Reports, Series P-23, No.153, *America's Centenarians*, (Data from the 1980 Census), U.S. Government Printing Office, Washington, D.C.

If we calculate the proportion (of those aged 100 and above among those aged 65 and above) for the 1980 enumerated U.S. white male population (.81), we find that the U.S. result is over five times as great as in Sweden (.14) or the Netherlands (.16). For the enumerated U.S. white female population, the calculated proportion for the U.S. was about four times greater than that of either European country. Comparing the US black populations to Sweden and the Netherlands, the results are even more exaggerated. Taking the number of enumerated black males (2,504) as a proportion of the black male population aged 65 and over (849,356) per 1,000 yields a proportion of 2.95. This result is over twenty-one times the proportion found in Sweden (.14). For black females, the calculated proportion of 3.61 is over eleven times greater than that found in Sweden (.31).

The Black-White Mortality Crossover

Life expectancy measures the average number of additional years a person would live if the present age-specific mortality rates of the population were to persist. Racial differences in life expectancy have long been observed in the United States, wherein black life expectancy at various ages is generally lower than that of whites. At the advanced ages, however, a reversal in life expectancy is observed whereby blacks have more years remaining on average than whites. In the official 1969-71 life tables from the National Center for Health Statistics, for instance, whites are expected to live .92 years longer than blacks. By age 75, however, blacks have .62 years longer to live than whites on average (NCHS, 1975). This phenomenon, which has been referred to as the racial mortality crossover, exists in both the male and the female populations, but is observed at different ages.

Two hypotheses have been advanced in attempts to interpret this mortality crossover. The first supposition, a biological selection argument, is a modified version of "survival of the fittest" theory. Those blacks who have survived the excessive environmental stresses of their younger years may be destined by natural selection to live an especially long life (U.S. Bureau of the Census, 1984a; McCord and Freeman, 1990). Manton refined this hypothesis by ascribing the crossover to the effect of differential mortality selection on a heterogeneous population. If individuals in populations are heterogeneous with respect to their endowment for longevity and/ or there are racial differences in the intrinsic rate of aging, then a crossover or convergence of the age-specific mortality rates of two populations can occur if one population has markedly higher earlier mortality (Manton, 1980, 1982; Manton, Stallard and Vaupel, 1979; Manton, Poss, and Wing, 1979; Manton and Poss, 1977; Manton and Stallard, 1981).

The first school implies that high mortality in the early ages is associated with low mortality later in life. This would require, however, that genetic susceptibilities to death in childhood be positively correlated with genetic susceptibilities to death in adulthood (Elo and Preston, 1991). This seems unlikely given the relatively small numbers of deaths ascribed to genetically-linked traits (Farley and Allen, 1987) and the different disease processes afflicting the two age groups (Farley and Allen, 1987; Elo and Preston, 1991). Furthermore, it has been argued that the relatively poor environment experienced by members of a disadvantaged cohort early in life is likely to persist as they age, causing high rather than low mortality later in life (Coale and Kisker, 1986). Numerous empirical studies support this positive relationship between early-life conditions and subsequent adult mortality. Kermack, McKendrick and McKinlay (1934a,b), in studies of British and Swedish death rates, concluded that environmental conditions during a cohort's first fifteen years of life determined the cohort's later adult mortality experience (Elo and Preston, 1991; Horn, 1985). Preston and van de Walle (1978) reached an analogous conclusion using historical data from urban France (See Elo and Preston, 1991, and Young, 1978, for detailed reviews of studies which relate early-life conditions to adult mortality). Evidence also exists which links specific childhood infectious agents (such as tuberculous) with conditions that can affect adult mortality. Hence, those exposed to these agents during the early ages could be expected to be more frail at the older ages than groups not imperiled by these diseases (Coale and Kisker, 1986). (See Elo and Preston, 1991, for detailed review of studies which relate specific infectious agents to adult mortality).

Murray, Khatib and Jackson (1989) speculate that early life conditions positively effect subsequent adult mortality for the U.S. black population. They argue that economic deprivation and racism, apparent throughout the life course of blacks, have caused poor nutritional status, inadequate housing, and poor health conditions combined with deficient access to adequate health care. These conditions continue into the older ages. Additional cohort-, race-, and sex-specific, empirical research is required to determine the magnitude of the relationship between childhood conditions and adult mortality experience in the United States.

The second school (Zelnik, 1969; Coale and Kisker, 1990; Preston et al., 1991) attributes the crossover to the questionable accuracy of the data sources at the advanced ages. Uncertainties about mortality conditions, which are particularly large for the black population, result from questions regarding the completeness of death registration, the quality of coverage in the censuses, and especially the quality of age reporting in all of the data sources (Preston et al., 1991). Critics, however, suggest that attributing the crossover to only measurement artifact is insufficient because: (1) partial adjustment for these factors has failed to eliminate the crossover (Kitagawa and Hauser, 1973; Manton, 1980, 1982; Rives, 1977, cited in Markides and Mindel, 1987; US Bureau of the Census, 1984a), (2) the crossover has been observed in both period and cohort data and over time in the same nation (Nam and Ockay, 1978), and, (3) the crossover has been observed in investigations less subject to data source inaccuracies (Wing et al., 1985; Kestenbaum, 1992).

In this book, the results of additional research will be presented on the role of data inconsistencies as related to the crossover phenomena. Before considering the absorbing question of why a racial mortality crossover exists at the advanced ages, it is first necessary to document that such a crossover truly exists.

A BRIEF DESCRIPTION OF FUTURE CHAPTERS

Chapter 2 will present an introductory evaluation of the quality of the three US decennial censuses (1970, 1980, and 1990) to be used in this book. Chapter 3 will provide analogous treatment of death registration and immigration statistics. These examinations, which will provide a detailed review of the literature, will focus on issues of completeness of coverage and misreporting of demographic characteristics for the older population in the official sources.

Chapter 4 will highlight a number of inherent problems in the particular data sources and will provide justification for adjustments to the official data. This chapter will focus on problems that are unique to the particular data source at a given time. Methodologies employed to modify the sources will also be discussed.

In Chapter 5, we describe a diagnostic intercensal cohort methodology which allows us to evaluate inconsistencies in the old-age census and death registration statistics.

Overview 11

The final chapter presents empirically-based ratios of observed population to expected population for the US white and US African American old-age populations for two intercensal periods, 1970-80 and 1980-90. The ratios are subsequently examined in light of evidence concerning the nature of coverage and content error in the basic data sources.

II

Quality of Decennial Census Data on the Older Population

This chapter provides a detailed review of previous evaluations of decennial US census statistics for the population aged 60 and above for years 1970, 1980, and 1990. The examination focuses on issues of completeness of coverage and misreporting of demographic characteristics for the older population in the official sources. While we believe that age misreporting is the predominant source of error in the official statistics, evaluation in this chapter will allow a preliminary test of the validity of that assumption. Further, the review affords justifications for modifications made to the official data utilized in this book.

Six major sections are presented in this chapter. The first presents background information relevant to all three of the censuses. The second describes the methods of evaluation used to judge the quality of the enumerations. The third, fourth, and fifth sections highlight the 1970, 1980, and 1990 censuses respectively. The final section briefly considers two specific data quality issues in the US censuses: the degree of age heaping and inconsistencies in the reporting of race.

BACKGROUND

The official, complete-count census enumerations refer to the resident population of the 50 states and the District of Columbia, with individuals generally counted at their usual place of residence on April 1. Included in the enumerations are (1) members of the Armed Forces living in the United States, (2) crews of merchant vessels that were berthed in a US port or inside the territorial waters of the United States, (3) the institutionalized population; (4) Americans travelling abroad temporarily, such as on vacation or on business, and, (5) foreign citizens having their usual residence (legally or illegally) in the US, including those working or studying in the United States, except foreign military and diplomatic personnel and their families who are living in embassies or similar quarters. Specifically excluded from the census enumerations of resident population are: (1) the populations of outlying areas of the United States, such as Puerto Rico, American Samoa, and Guam. (Note, however, that while these populations are excluded from enumerations of the resident population, separate publications detailing demographic, social, and economic characteristics of these populations are published by the US Bureau of the Census), (2) Americans overseas for an extended period, e.g., military personnel overseas, crews of merchant vessels outside of US territorial waters, US civilian citizens resident overseas, and US students attending foreign universities, (3) foreign citizens temporarily visiting the United States, and, (4) foreign citizens living on the grounds of an embassy. The official statistics do not adjust for census undercount, e.g. the failure to find and enumerate legal residents and undocumented immigrants.

The term "resident population" implies that both the legal population and undocumented immigrants are included in the census tabulations. While some undocumented persons were likely to have been residing in the US at the time of the 1970 census, it appears that only a negligible number were counted. Hence, the legal resident population approximated the total resident population in the 1970 census. In the 1980 count, however, the US Bureau of the Census estimates that, for the first time ever, a significant number of undocumented persons were counted. Estimates indicate that the count equalled 2.06 million undocumented persons. Of this number, in the age group 60 and above, 10,000 white males were enumerated; 19,000 white females; 3,000 black males; and 6,000 black females (US Bureau of the Census, 1988). Woodrow-Lafield (1995) reports that at least 2.1-2.4 million undocumented residents were enumerated in the 1990 census. Further, she reports that the number of unenumerated undocumented residents may easily range between 0.5 million and 3.0 million. Estimates by age were not reported.

In the censuses, individuals' sex, race, and age characteristics are described primarily through self-reporting. In cases of missing or inconsistent data, however, the Census Bureau assigns acceptable entries through an allocation procedure. First, attempts are made to deduce missing values based on other characteristics reported for the same individual. If unsuccessful, a value is assigned in such a way as

Quality of the Decennial Census Data on the Older Population 15

to insure that the distribution of characteristics in the enumerated population is maintained. The same procedures are used in all censuses, except where noted.

To assign a value for an individual's sex, attempts are first made to determine gender based on the individual's given name and reported household relationship. If this procedure fails, an entry for the person is assigned that is consistent with entries for other persons with similar characteristics.

Race, as reported to the Census Bureau, represents self-categorization by individuals, as opposed to a genetically-based designation of biological origin. If a race value was missing, initial attempts focused on assignment of race based on the race of other household members. If unavailable for any household member, the race of the head of the preceding household processed was assigned. It must be noted that the Census Bureau changed its procedure between 1970 and 1980 for assigning race for persons of mixed parentage who did not respond to the race question. For the 1970 census, for persons of mixed parentage who did not provide a single response to the race question, the Census Bureau allocated the race of the person's father. For the 1980 census, however, the race of the individual's mother was utilized. The impact of the procedural change is most consequential at younger ages.

Age refers to age in completed years on April 1 of the census year. Respondents in 1970 and 1980 were requested to provide their month and year of birth in a form that was readable by FOSDIC (Film Optical Sensing Device for Input to Computer). For most items on the census questionnaire, the information supplied by the respondent was indicated by marking the answers in predesignated positions that would be optically "read" by FOSDIC from a microfilm copy of the questionnaire and transferred onto magnetic computer tape with no intervening manual processing. Data on age was then calculated by the computer by subtracting the date of birth from the census date. Respondents had also been asked to print their age at last birthday as well as their month and year of birth. These entries, which were not in a machine-readable form, were utilized only during the review process to assign values to missing FOSDIC-readable responses. Only age (last birthday) and year of birth were requested in the 1990 census. Question #5 asked the respondents to both write out and provide FOSDIC-readable responses for the two entries.

As shown in Table 2.1, the percent of allocation by various demographic characteristics for the total population had remained fairly constant in the 1970 and 1980 censuses. Increases in the allocation of sex and race are observed in the 1990 census.

Table 2.1

Percentage of Total Enumerated Population for which Demographic Characteristics were Allocated; US Censuses: 1970, 1980, and 1990

Characteristic	Census Year		
	1970	1980	1990
Sex	0.9%	0.8%	1.2%
Race	1.5	1.5	2.1
Age (all ages)	2.7	2.9	2.5
(65 & over)	3.6	4.0	NA

Notes: (1) The term "allocation" means that a characteristic was assigned in the absence of machine-readable entry or changed to make consistent with other entries during the computer editing, (2) universe: persons not substituted, (3) NA: not available, (4) the table is based on *official* statistics from the US Bureau of the Census, which do not include modification for race and/or age problems identified in the 1980 and 1990 censuses.

Sources: (1) US Bureau of the Census. 1972a. *General Population Characteristics*. 1970 Census of Population and Housing, Final Report PC(1)-B1. United States Summary. Washington, D.C.: US Government Printing Office. Table B-1. (2) -----. 1983a. *General Population Characteristics*. 1980 Census of Population and Housing, Final Report PC80-1-B1. United States Summary. Washington, D.C.: US Government Printing Office. (3) -----. 1992. *Summary Tape File 1C*. 1990 Census of Population and Housing. US Summary. Compact Disk: CD90-1C.

In the 1970 and 1980 censuses, assignment of age by the Census Bureau was positively correlated with age. In the 1970 census, age was allocated for 2.7% of the total population but, for the population 65 and over, age was allocated for 3.6%. In 1980, overall allocation of age was 2.9%, whereas allocation for the aged population increased to 4.0%. The US Bureau of the Census (1976; 1984) further

Quality of the Decennial Census Data on the Older Population 17

notes that, while about 10% of all persons whose ages were reported in the 1970 and 1980 censuses were aged 65 and over, about 14.0% of the allocated ages fell into this age group. Allocation of age is also known to have caused an exaggeration in the count of centenarians in the 1980 census. The Census Bureau (1987b) notes that "difficulties with the procedures used in the allocation of age allowed an estimated 25 percent inflation in the tabulations for the population 100 and over." Over 32,000 centenarians were reported in official 1980 census statistics. Of this number, 24,000 self-reported an age of 100 or over, whereas the remaining 8,000 were so allocated (US Bureau of the Census, 1984a).

A procedural change in the allocation procedures for assignment of age was introduced for the 1990 census. A conscious decision was made to minimize the assignment of individuals to rare ages although it was recognized that certain discontinuities with previous censuses would ensue (Hollmann and Spencer, 1992a). Hollmann and Spencer (ibid) cite numerical examples of some of the changes in procedures between 1980 and 1990. Referring to persons in the 1990 census:

> 45,000 people gave a year of birth of 1874 to 1890 and an age of 0 to 16. Under 1980 rules they were all 99 to 115; under 1990 rules they are 0 to 16.

> 100,000 children who were not at least 6 years younger than their oldest parent were made 18 to 44 years younger.

> 105,000 people said that they were born before 1904, but their age was inconsistent. In 1980 they were 85 to 115; in 1990 their age was accepted.

> 20,000 people said they were born in 1900, but their age was not 89 or 90. Under 1980 rules they were made 89 or 90. In 1990 their age was accepted.

> 61,000 parents were less than 15 years older than the younger of their adult child and the child's spouse. In 1980 they were made old enough most of the time; in 1990 their age was retained and their relationship was changed.

52,000 people who were born in 1990 reported an age of 2+. Under 1980 rules they would be age 0. In 1990 they were 2+.

145,000 people said they were born since 1973 and gave an inconsistent age. They also said they were ever-married or gave an adult relationship such as spouse. In 1980 most would have been under 15 and had their other characteristics made consistent. In 1990 their age over 15 was kept.

87,000 "children" were turned into spouses in 1990 and their adult age kept. In 1980 they were left as children and many were made younger. (Hollmann and Spencer, 1992a).

GENERAL METHODS FOR EVALUATING CENSUS COVERAGE AND CONTENT ERRORS

Various sources of error exist in the decennial censuses. Completeness of coverage refers to the degree to which the census accurately counts all individuals included in its enumeration frame. Errors in coverage can arise from the unintentional exclusion of individuals or of households, duplicate counting of individuals, and erroneous inclusion of persons not in the enumeration frame.

A second general category of error is content error, or flaws in the demographic characteristics reported for persons who were enumerated in the census. Two types of content error are particularly consequential for this study, the misreporting of age and the misreporting of race.

As discussed in Chapter 1, age misreporting refers to the intentional or inadvertent introduction of errors into reported age data. Inconsistencies in the reporting of race can also introduce appreciable errors. Demographic analysis relies upon statistics from various sources, including prior censuses, the vital registration system, Medicare enrollments, etc. Differences in the reporting of race among the various sources would lead to classification errors in the estimates. Two sources of inconsistency in race classification exist: (1) categorization of children of mixed race parents, and, (2) variations in the reporting of race by adults over time, particularly for the black race group (Robinson and Lapham, 1991). Empirical evidence on

Quality of the Decennial Census Data on the Older Population 19

racial identification in the US 1970-1990 censuses by the US black population will be presented later in this chapter.

Disparate evaluation methods can be utilized to analyze the quality of the decennial censuses. Techniques of demographic analysis allow construction of estimates of the total US population and its components by race, sex, and age group from data that are independent of the particular census. Such aggregate data sources include historical statistics on births, deaths, immigration, emigration, past censuses, Medicare enrollments, expected sex ratios, and life tables.

For instance, one demographic method of estimating a cohort's size is through the basic demographic accounting equation:

$$P_I = B - D + I - E \qquad (2.1)$$

where P_1 is the estimated size of the cohort at time 1, B is births, D represents deaths, I is immigration and E is emigration. For example, the estimate of the population aged 70 on April 1, 1990 is based on births from April 1919 to March 1920, reduced by deaths to the single-year cohort in each year between birth and 1990, and adjusted for net immigration over the 70 year period.

Demographic methods depend on the logical consistency of the various kinds of demographic data in order to derive an expected or corrected population for comparison with the census figures (US Bureau of the Census, 1974). While demographic analysis is generally accepted as providing the best measures of the coverage of the total population and of net census errors for age-race-sex groups (US Bureau of the Census, 1974), the analytic techniques have limitations as well. While the method is undoubtedly capable of providing estimates of net error, it fails to provide information on its components (incorrect inclusion or duplication of individuals, exclusion of persons, misreporting of demographic characteristics). Similarly, while the approach shows inconsistencies between different sources of data, identification of the data set in error or distribution of the error between the sets is impossible. A further liability is that the techniques require reasonably complete component data (such as vital and immigration statistics). Component data with content or coverage deficiencies can be adjusted, but the result of assuming a pattern or magnitude of bias in the components is the increased probability of introducing bias into the calculated demographic estimates.

A second important evaluation method is to examine individual records from the census against an independent source. The Census Bureau has matched its records with Medicare files, reinterview questionnaires, and the Current Population Survey (an ongoing national survey of the civilian, noninstitutionalized population that is conducted monthly by the Census Bureau for the US Bureau of Labor Statistics). The principal advantage of record check evaluation is its ability to provide estimates of gross error (erroneous inclusions, omissions, and characteristic misreporting). However, a number of problems are apparent. First, in general, the investigations are clearly able to highlight differences in the reporting of characteristics between the two sources, but are unable to judge which source (if either) is accurate. Second, these methods generally are based on samples of records, and as such may be affected by sampling error or random variability. A third limitation is the possibility of selectivity bias introduced by the inability to match all individuals in the two data sources. If the response error distributions of the unmatched persons differed from those matched, we could expect bias. Fourth, the same types of persons may be excluded from both data systems, leading to correlation bias. And, finally, as mentioned by Robinson and Lapham (1991), a limitation of many match studies undertaken by the Census Bureau is that they evaluate inconsistencies between two data sets at a point in time, not cohort changes in reporting over time.

EVALUATION OF THE 1970 CENSUS

Official tabulations of the 1970 population by basic demographic characteristics are presented in *Series B--US Summary of the 1970 Census* (US Bureau of the Census, 1972a). By "demographic characteristics", we refer to age (single years to 84, five-year groupings to 99, and open-ended at age 100), race (black/white), and sex (male/female). Although these numbers are widely used by researchers, they are known to contain certain errors.

The most serious problem for our investigation is the conspicuous overstatement of the number of persons aged 100 years or more. Major discrepancies in the enumerated centenarian population have been identified for both sexes and for all race groupings (Siegel, 1974; Siegel and Passel, 1976; US Bureau of the Census, 1974). Whereas the census counted 106,441 centenarians, indirect demographic estimates indicated that the correct centenarian count should have been in the range of 3,000-8,000, with a preferred estimate of 4,800. Over-estimation of centenarians in censuses conducted prior to 1970 are believed to have resulted primarily from age misstatements by respondents, but the authors attribute the large discrepancy in the 1970 census to the manner in which the age question appeared on the census form and to processing errors associated with the age question. Because the overcount resulted from misinterpretation of the census form, the accurate ages are believed to be spread over the entire age scale. Approximately 10,000 of the excess centenarians are estimated to be between the ages of 65 and 99 (US Bureau of the Census, 1973), and, as mentioned, about 4,800 are believed to be true centenarians.

Siegel and Passel (1976) employed various demographic techniques to reach this conclusion, including: (1) comparison with Medicare records, (2) forward survival of the 1960 and 1950 populations using either life table or Medicare rates, and (3) population reconstruction using either a stationary population assumption or least squares estimation techniques. The alternative estimates of the centenarian population by sex and race are presented in Table 3.3 of this book. Discussion of the quality of the estimates is further provided in Siegel and Passel (ibid).

A second problem is the result of misclassification of the population by race in the complete-count tabulations. Specifically, the "white" category in 1970 was intended to include persons who self-identified their race as white, as well as persons who wrote-in a distinctive entry that suggested Indo-European stock, such as Polish, Mexican or Bulgarian. The "black" category should have included persons who indicated their race as black or Negro, as well as persons who wrote-in entries such as Jamaican, Nigerian or West Indian. However, some individuals with the above write-in entries were incorrectly classified as members of the "other races" category for the Series B tabulations, since not all were identified and corrected before the 100% processing (US Bureau of the Census, 1972a). For the Series C (US Bureau of the Census, 1972b) sample tabulations, an editing process transferred 327,000 persons (or about 63% of the total population of "unspecified races") from the "other races" category to the "white" category. Of these numbers, 21,000 persons aged 65+ were transferred. Since the effect on the "black" classification was inconsequential, no adjustment was made.

Finally, the official 1970 legal resident population count for the United States is 203,235,298, as opposed to 203,211,926 as presented in the Series B statistics. The difference, over 23,000, represents corrections for errors in the population counts of local areas which were discovered after the initial tabulations were published (US Bureau of the Census, 1974).

Additional coverage and content errors are evident in the 1970 census. Assessment of the quality of the census data was undertaken by the Census Bureau in three major studies, each employing a different evaluation method. The following paragraphs provide brief descriptions of the evaluations. Detailed discussion of each of the studies is provided later in this chapter.

The first study (US Bureau of the Census, 1974), was designed to estimate net coverage error employing the method of demographic analysis. Detailed presentation of the results obtained and discussion of the limitations of the estimates is presented later.

A second study (US Bureau of the Census, 1973) decomposed the components of the net error through a record check study in which a sample from the Medicare enrollment files (adjusted for under-enrollment) was matched with census records. The analysis allowed estimation of the extent of gross exclusion of persons aged 65 years and above from the census as well as appraisal of the degree of duplication of such persons. Data on differences in age misreporting between the census and Medicare were also reported.

To evaluate content error, a third study (US Bureau of the Census, 1975) matched individual records from the 1970 census 20 percent sample with the March 1970 CPS (Current Population Survey). The Census-CPS match study allowed analysis of response variability for demographic characteristics (such as age, race, and sex) by persons who were enumerated in both data collection systems. The study was based on matches for 6,864 households, representing 21,502 persons (US Bureau of the Census, 1975). In the 1970 census-CPS study, 75.2% of the maximum "in-scope" households were successfully matched (US Bureau of the Census, ibid). Detailed discussion of the findings for the aged population is presented later in this section, paying particular attention to the limitations of the estimates.

The section concludes with a summary analysis of the quality of the 1970 census.

Evaluation of 1970 Census using Demographic Methods

The US Bureau of the Census (1974) employed demographic analysis to estimate net census error (which includes errors of coverage and of age misreporting) in the 1970 census statistics. For the evaluation of the aged population, four sets of alternative estimates based on different methodologies were calculated. The preferred set of estimates (Table 2.2) are based on a composite of data sources, analytic methods, and assumptions. For the aged population (aged 65 and above), the estimates of the population are based on Medicare enrollments and expected sex ratios. For age group 35 to 64, estimates are derived from a variety of sources, including (1) expected sex ratios, (2) Coale-Zelnik (1963) white estimates for 1950, and, (3) Coale-Rives (1973) black estimates for 1960.

Table 2.2
Preferred Estimates of Net Underenumeration, in Absolute Numbers and Percent: 1970 Census, by Sex, Race, and Age

	Undercount (in Thousands)			
	Whites		Blacks	
Age	Males	Females	Males	Females
All Ages	2,186	1,283	1,181	695
55-59 years	93	60	49	42
60-64 years	86	115	25	23
65-69 years	-5	-38	-25	-44
70-74 years	-2	12	-4	14
75 years & over	101	270	9	69
65 years & over	93	243	-20	38

Table 2.2 (continued)

Net Underenumeration (in Percent)

Age	Whites Males	Whites Females	Blacks Males	Blacks Females	Difference Blacks-Whites Males	Difference Blacks-Whites Females
Total	2.5	1.4	9.9	5.5	7.4	4.1
55-59	2.1	1.3	10.9	8.2	8.8	6.9
60-64	2.3	2.7	7.0	5.5	4.7	2.8
65-69	-0.2	-1.1	-10.1	-14.5	-9.9	-13.4
70-74	-0.1	0.4	-2.2	5.6	-2.1	5.2
75+	3.6	5.9	4.3	19.0	0.7	13.1
65+	1.2	2.2	-3.1	4.2	-4.3	2.0

Notes: (1) Refers to the resident population, (2) Base of percents is corresponding estimate of corrected population, (3) Estimates have been adjusted for race misclassification in the complete count, affecting some 327,000 persons, mostly of Spanish ancestry, and for a gross overstatement of the centenarian population, amounting to about 103,000 persons. See text for details, (4) A minus indicates a net overcount, (5) Preferred estimates, as presented, are based on a composite of analytic methods.

Source: Extracted from: US Bureau of the Census. 1974. *Estimates of coverage of the population by sex, race, and age: demographic analysis.* 1970 Census of Population and Housing: Evaluation & Research Program, PHC(E)-4. By J.S. Siegel. Washington, DC: US GPO. Tables 4-6.

Although the coverage estimates for the population aged 65 and over show modest error rates of 4.2% or less for each of the race-sex groups, such aggregation tends to obscure critical differences. Referring to Table 2.2, which presents the preferred set of estimates, for most ages, the combination of net coverage error and net age misreporting error results in a net census undercount. For all race-sex groups aged 65-69 and for all males aged 70-74, however, the estimates suggest a net overcount, which can occur only as the result of gross duplication of individuals, erroneous inclusion of persons who were not in the enumeration frame, or from age misreporting. The large undercounts, particularly for blacks, in the age groups 55-59 and 60-64 raise the possibility that members of these age groups have incorrectly reported their ages as 65 and above.

The net error rate for blacks exceeded that of whites in each sex-age group. The absolute difference was particularly substantial for females in the age categories 65-69 and 75 years and older. At age 65-69, a net overcount of 1.1% was estimated for white females, whereas the corresponding estimate for the black female population was 14.5%, a difference of 13.4%. At ages 75 and over, white females were under-counted by 5.9% compared to black females with an undercount rate of 19.0%, a difference of 13.1%.

In most cases, the net error rate for females exceeded that of males, but the differential was of a smaller magnitude than in the racial differences discussed above.

Underenumeration at ages 75 and above are particularly large when compared to younger ages, particularly for black females with an undercount estimate of 19.0%.

The Census Bureau (1974) notes, however, that the estimates of coverage of the white population are more reliable than the comparable black population estimates because of better quality and greater volume of data available for the evaluation and the more limited scope of the assumptions employed. It is further suggested that there is uncertainty not only about the magnitude of the error rate but also about its direction for the black aged population (US Bureau of the Census, ibid). This results from different estimation outcomes to the alternative demographic procedures applied to the black data. For illustrative purposes, refer to Table 2.3, which presents alternative estimates of the percent of net undercount of the black, female population.

Table 2.3

Alternative Estimates derived by Demographic Analysis of Percent Net Undercount of the Black Female Population: US, 1970 Census

Age	Set A	Set B	Set C	Preferred Set D
All Ages	6.8	6.1	4.8	5.5
55-59 years	9.7	9.7	9.8	8.2
60-64 years	12.6	12.6	8.5	5.5
65-69 years	-9.7	-14.5	-1.5	-14.5
70-74 years	-0.9	5.6	0.4[1]	5.6
75 and over	34.2	19.0	NA	19.0
65 and over	12.0	4.2	-0.3	4.2

Notes: [1]Refers to ages 70 and above. *Set A* estimates use forward projection techniques, based on corrected population of 1960; *Set B* estimates, which are a partial variant of Set A estimates, introduce data for the corrected aged population based on tabulations of Medicare enrollments; *Set C* estimates are based on a set of estimates of coverage of the native black population by Coale and Rives (1973); *Set D* estimates, the preferred set, are an aggregation of the data, methods, and assumptions implemented in Sets A, B, and C.

Source: extracted from US Bureau of the Census. 1974. *Estimates of coverage of population by sex, race, and age: demographic analysis.* 1970 Census of Population and Housing: Evaluation and Research Program, PHC(E)-4. By J.S. Siegel. Washington, DC: US Government Printing Office. Tables 5-6.

It should be mentioned that recent unpublished undercount estimates produced by the US Bureau of the Census for the 1970 census differ from all four sets of estimates presented in US Bureau of the Census (1974). While the magnitudes of the undercount estimates vary in the updated statistics, the general patterns observed in the preferred set of 1974 are maintained.

As previously mentioned, a limitation of demographic analysis in the evaluation of census data is that it fails to partition net error into its sources. Such components of error include the omission of individuals, overenumeration (or duplication) of persons, and distortion caused by misreporting of demographic characteristics, such as age, race, and sex.

Evaluation of 1970 Census by Record Matching with Medicare Records

Another US Bureau of the Census evaluation report (1973) attempts to decompose the components of the net error for the aged population. This was accomplished through a record check study in which a sample of persons enrolled in Medicare were matched to their 1970 census records. No check was made in the opposite direction, i.e. there was no attempt to find Census respondents in the Medicare files. Using the Medicare records as the standard, the authors attempted to estimate the percent of persons missed by the census, the percent double-counted, and the amount of age, sex, and race misreporting. Four independent evaluations were carried out: (a) for the white, male population with a sample size equal to 3,945; (b) for white females with a sample size of 2,415; (c) for males in the "black and other races" category with sample size equal to 972; and, (d) for females in the "black and other races category" with sample size of 1,081. While separate analysis of the black population was not carried out, blacks make up a large proportion of the nonwhite population aged 60 and above. Of the 2,547,234 individuals (both sexes) enumerated in the nonwhite population in the given age range, 90.0 percent (2,292,531) were classified as black (US Bureau of the Census, 1972).

The results of these evaluations are not directly comparable to the results of the demographic analysis for three reasons. First, the Medicare records were matched with the official, 100% count census data referred to as the Series B tabulations. Hence, the matched census record was adjusted for neither the centenarian nor the race classification problems. Second, the Medicare record study did not search records for persons aged under 65 years. Hence, the extent to which such persons reported their age as 65 or more in the census was not measurable (US Bureau of the Census, 1973). Third, the record study attempted to measure specific components of error, as opposed to the demographic study in which net error was addressed. Note also that the record check study is based on a sample, and as such is subject to sampling variability.

Table 2.4 presents the gross missed rate for all persons aged 65 and over for the record study. The gross missed rate is intended to describe only one source of error, i.e. gross omissions from the census. It is calculated by estimating the number of sample persons who were missed in the census per 100 enumerated in the same census. Overall, the gross missed rate for all persons aged 65 and over was estimated to be 4.9%, but varied by age, by sex, and by race. The rate appears to be positively correlated with age, in that the missed rate generally increased as age increased. For the total population, the missed rate for ages 65-69 was 3.5%; at ages 70-74, it was estimated that 5.2% were missed; and for ages 75 and above, 5.8% were omitted. The missed rate for persons 75 and over exceeded the rate for those 65-74 and the amount of difference was beyond what might be due to sampling variability at the 95 percent confidence level (Census Bureau, ibid).

The estimated gross missed rates further indicated that males were more likely to be omitted than females. For the total population aged 65 and above, males were missed 5.7% of the time, whereas the female missed rate was 4.4%. This difference was observed for each of the four race-sex combinations and for each of the elderly age groupings.

A final observation about the estimated gross missed rates for persons aged 65 and over is that the coverage was better for whites than for the "black and other races" category. The total aged white population was omitted 4.4% of the time, compared to a gross missed rate of 11.0% for the total aged black and other races population. The wide differences were noted for each of the age groups. Special attention should be drawn to the estimates for males of the "black and other races" category. The estimated gross missed rates for this group are especially large (12.6% or over) for each of the age categories, and reach a high of 15.0% for age group 70-74. Members of this group were missed about 2.5 times the rate for white males.

Table 2.4

Estimated Gross Missed Rates[1] in the 1970 Census based on Medicare Record Check for Persons Aged 65 and Over, by Age, Race, and Sex

Age and Sex	Whites Missed Rate	Whites Standard Error	Blacks Missed Rate	Blacks Standard Error
Both Sexes:				
65-69 years	3.0	0.7	9.5	1.2
70-74 years	4.7	0.6	9.9	1.2
75+ years	5.3	0.5	13.4	1.3
Males:				
65-69 years	4.0	0.6	12.6	1.9
70-74 years	4.8	0.7	15.0	2.3
75+ years	5.8	0.7	13.6	2.1
Females:				
65-69 years	2.1	0.6	6.7	1.4
70-74 years	4.6	0.9	6.5	1.4
75+ years	5.0	0.7	13.3	1.7

Notes: [1]Missed rates are an estimate of the number of missed persons per 100 divided by the number of persons enumerated in the census.

Source: US Bureau of the Census. 1973. *The Medicare record check: an evaluation of the coverage of persons 65 years of age and over in the 1970 Census.* 1970 Census of Population & Housing: Evaluation & Research Program, PHC(E)-7. Washington, DC: US Govt. Printing Office. Table 1.

The record study also evaluated the extent of over-enumeration in the aged 1970 census population. A sub-sample (1/3) of the Medicare sample was asked to provide other addresses where they might also have been enumerated in the census. A search of the census records for the alternative addresses was then undertaken. Only two sample persons were found to be duplicated in the census. Allowing for sampling error (at the 95% confidence interval) the maximum amount of overenumeration in the census for the population aged 65 and over is trivial, estimated to be less than one-sixth of one percent (US Bureau of the Census, ibid).

The Medicare-Census match also allowed estimation of age misreporting in the Census, again assuming that the Medicare records are a viable benchmark against which to judge the census records. The authors note that "the results of the comparisons suggest that age misreporting in the census for persons 65 and over may be large enough to introduce appreciable distortions in demographic coverage estimates for 5-year age groups" (US Bureau of the Census, 1973).

Estimates of the consistency of age reporting (for 5-year age groups) between the census record and the Medicare file for persons aged 65+ in the Medicare sample were calculated by the Census Bureau. Two measures were estimated to characterize the degree of age misreporting. The first, the "index of inconsistency" describes response variance or the gross differences between the two sources on a scale from 0 (perfect consistency) to 100 (complete inconsistency). Estimates of reporting accuracy are computed from entries in a table similar to Table 2.5:

	Table 2.5		
	Census Records		
Medicare Records	In Category	Out of Category	Total
In Category	a	b	np_2
Out of Category	c	d	nq_2
Total	np_1	nq_1	n
Source: US Bureau of the Census. 1973. *The Medicare record check: an evaluation of the coverage of persons 65 years of age and over in the 1970 census.* 1970 Census of Population: Evaluation and Research Program. PHC(E)-7. Washington, DC: US Government Printing Office.			

Quality of the Decennial Census Data on the Older Population 31

The methodology to compute the index of inconsistency is presented in US Bureau of the Census (1974) as follows:

$$I = \frac{b+c}{n\,(p_1 q_2 + p_2 q_1)}, \quad (2.2),$$

where,
a and d are Medicare and census data that are consistent;
b and c are inconsistent data; and,
n is the size of the particular sample.

p_1 and q_1 are, respectively, the proportions of cases that are in and out of the category according to the census, and p_2 and q_2 relate to the same classification according to Medicare.

In general, values less than 20 indicate a low degree of inconsistency, indices between 20 and 50 suggest moderate inconsistency, and values above 50 evidence high degrees of inconsistency. Related to this index is the "L-fold index", which is simply a weighted average for distributions with more than two categories.

The second measure, the "net difference rate", measures net error. It describes the dissimilarities between the Census and the Medicare sources in the percent in category. If the proportion is larger in the Census, the net difference rate will be positive. A negative value denotes that the proportion is larger in the Medicare file. The net difference rate is computed from Table 2.5 as:

$$NDR = \frac{c-b}{n} \quad (2.3)$$

Table 2.6 presents the indices of age-reporting errors in the 1970 Census for persons aged 65 and over based on the Medicare record check. As evidenced by the table, the net difference rates are notably below the index of inconsistency values and often fail to be significantly different than zero. This is not surprising in that this measure gauges the extent of net error. The rate can be suppressed by the balancing effects of age misreporting into and out of each age group, and by the relatively small and stable characteristics of the percent of total population in any age classification (US Bureau of the Census, 1975).

Table 2.6

Indices of Age-Reporting Errors in the 1970 Census for Persons Aged 65 and Over, Based on Medicare Record Check, (expressed as percents)

Age in Medicare	Index of Inconsistency (I)	95% Confidence Interval for I	Percent in Class, Medicare	Net Difference Rate (NDR)	95% Confidence Interval for NDR
White Males					
65-69	1.5	1.0 to 2.2	36.1	0.2	-0.1 to 0.5
70-74	3.3	2.4 to 4.4	27.4	0.0	-0.4 to 0.4
75+	1.7	1.2 to 2.5	36.6	-0.5	-0.8 to -0.2
L-fold index, all cat.	2.3	1.8 to 3.1			
White Females					
65-69	4.7	3.5 to 6.3	30.1	0.2	0.2 to 1.4
70-74	9.0	7.1 to 11.3	25.0	0.4	-0.4 to 1.2
75+	5.0	3.8 to 6.5	44.8	-1.7	
L-fold index, all cat.	6.4	5.2 to 7.9			-2.4 to -1.0

Table 2.6 (*continued*)

Black & Other, Males			
65-69	12.5	9.3 to 16.7	0.6	-1.1 to 2.4
70-74	23.2	18.4 to 29.1	-0.8	-3.0 to 1.5
75+	16.1	12.1 to 21.1	-2.0	-3.9 to -0.1
L-fold index, all cat.	18.3	15.2 to 22.2		
Black & Other, Females			
65-69	23.6	19.6 to 28.5	4.6	2.5 to 6.8
70-74	34.4	29.4 to 40.4	-3.0	-5.5 to -0.5
75+	22.1	18.2 to 26.9	-5.2	-7.2 to -3.1
L-fold index, all cat.	28.3	24.9 to 32.5		

Notes: (1) Sample excluded individuals with a Medicare age of less than 65 years, (2) Values for the index of inconsistency (I) can range from 0 (perfect consistency) to 100 (complete lack of consistency). I is a measure of gross error, (3) For the net difference rate (NDR), a positive value indicates that the proportion in category is larger in Census; a negative indicates that the proportion is larger in Medicare. The NDR is a measure of net error.

Source: US Bureau of the Census, 1973. Tables 58, 68, 78, and 88.

The results indicate that whites (of both sexes and in all age categories) had a low degree of inconsistency, with the index of inconsistency equal to or less than 9.0 in all cases. The black and other races category, in contrast, showed a higher degree of inconsistency, with the index ranging between 12.5 and 34.4. Females of this race category exhibited large values which indicated moderate inconsistency in all of the age groups. Females showed more inconsistency than males in all age groups and for both races.

For age group 65-69, the net difference rate was found to be positive, indicating that the proportion enumerated in that age category in the census exceeded those counted in Medicare. This conclusion is consistent with our interpretation of the results from the demographic evaluation, e.g. that persons correctly aged 60-64 reported into the 65-69 age group in the 1970 census. For the male populations, however, the results must be viewed with caution since the 95% confidence interval overlaps both positive and negative values in the Medicare study.

Age group 75 years and older is striking in that more persons were enumerated in the Medicare file than in the Census in each of the four race-sex groups. According to the authors, the explanation is that persons whose correct age is 75 and over reported themselves at younger ages in the census (US Bureau of the Census, 1973). Another compatible interpretation is that the Medicare file becomes less effective as a benchmark against which to judge census data at the oldest ages due to a higher rate of misreporting in the Medicare records among the first entrants.

In addition to the general errors associated with matching studies (discussed earlier), a number of problems with the specific Medicare-Census study are apparent. First, the investigation assumes the accuracy of characteristics reported in the Medicare file and uses such information as a benchmark against which to judge the Census data. Medicare data are generally believed to be of superior quality because persons enrolling in the program are required to provide verification of age. However, it appears that early enrollees who were well above the age of 65 at the time of the program's inception in 1966 were excused from providing a proof of age. The objective of the early program age verification was simply to ascertain whether an individual had attained age 65 (Coale and Kisker, 1990; Siegel and Passel, 1976). Incidental indications suggest that some of these persons were registered with exaggerated ages. Second, the study failed to include persons aged 65 or younger in the Medicare files. This seriously limits interpretation of the gross transfer of persons between age group 60-64 and older groups due to age misreporting.

Evaluation of Census Estimates based on Matching of a Census Sample with the CPS

A final study matched records of individuals enumerated in both the 1970 census 20% sample and the March 1970 CPS. Its purpose was to evaluate the accuracy of characteristics reported by these persons using indices of inconsistency and net difference rates.

The net difference rate was used to measure the absolute difference between the census proportion in category and the CPS proportion of persons in the same category. As such, it is a gauge of the amount of net errors or response bias in the sources. As evidenced by Table 2.7, the net difference rates are notably below the index of inconsistency values and fail to be significantly different than zero for any of the age-race-sex groups. As before, this can be explained: (1) by the equalizing effects of age misreporting into and out of each age group, and, (2) by the relatively small and stable characteristics of the percent of total population in any age classification (US Bureau of the Census, 1975).

To evaluate gross error, indices of inconsistency (using equation 2.2) were calculated. For the aged white population, the index ranged from 7 to 11, which indicates a low level of inconsistency. The black population in the same age categories, however, exhibited a higher degree of inconsistency with the index ranging from 15 to 19. Differentials were also noted between sexes, with the female population subject to slightly higher indices of inconsistency in each of the aged categories, except at ages 75 years and older.

Note that the index of inconsistency methodology used by the Census Bureau condensed age into five-year age groups with the open-ended interval beginning at age 75. The broad groupings can be expected to mask age misreporting within the age groupings. For instance, if an individual is reported at age 70 in the Census and at age 74 in the CPS, this discrepancy will not be discerned by the methods used. This may explain some of the unexpectedly low values for the index of inconsistency at ages 75 and above (Table 2.7: whites; females).

Table 2.7

Indices Measuring the Consistency between the March 1970 CPS and the 1970 Census 20-percent Sample: Age by Race

Age & Race	Index of Inconsistency (I)	95% Confidence Interval for I	Percent in Class	Net Difference Rate (NDR)	95% Confidence Interval for NDR
Whites					
60-64 years	10	8.0 to 11.2	4.1	0.0	-0.2 to 0.1
65-69 years	11	9.6 to 13.3	3.5	-0.1	-0.2 to 0.1
70-74 years	10	8.0 to 11.7	2.9	0.1	0.0 to 0.2
75 and over	7	5.6 to 8.6	3.4	0.1	0.0 to 0.2
Blacks					
60-64 years	18	12.2 to 27.1	3.8	0.2	-0.4 to 0.7
65-69 years	18	11.4 to 27.7	3.2	-0.1	-0.6 to 0.4
70-74 years	15	8.3 to 28.8	1.8	0.0	-0.4 to 0.4
75 and over	19	11.6 to 31.3	2.2	0.2	-0.2 to 0.7

Table 2.7 (continued): Age by Sex

Males			
60-64 years	8	6.4 to 10.8	-0.2 to 0.1
65-69 years	10	8.1 to 13.4	-0.2 to 0.2
70-74 years	9	6.9 to 12.4	-0.1 to 0.1
75 and over	9	6.5 to 11.5	0.0 to 0.3
Females			
60-64 years	12	9.7 to 14.2	-0.2 to 0.2
65-69 years	12	10.2 to 15.1	-0.3 to 0.1
70-74 years	11	8.7 to 13.9	0.0 to 0.3
75 and over	7	5.8 to 9.7	-0.1 to 0.2

Source: US Bureau of the Census. 1975. *Accuracy of data for selected population characteristics as measured by the 1970 CPS-Census Match.* 1970 Census of Population and Housing: Evaluation and Research Program. PHC(E)-11. Washington, D.C.: US Government Printing Office. Table 11.

Note: Data are restricted to persons with the same racial classification in CPS and census.

Summary Evaluation: Quality of Old-Age Population Statistics in the 1970 Census

National-level estimates of the coverage of the aged population in the 1970 census were presented in this section. These estimates were derived by various techniques, including demographic analysis, matching with administrative (Medicare) records, and matching with CPS records. A number of general conclusions for the old-age population can be inferred based on the evaluation studies. First, the magnitude of net error in the old-age statistics is greater than for the younger population. Second, although females exhibited higher net error rates as a result of higher levels of age misreporting, female net error rates were dampened by lower relative (to males) gross omission rates. Third, patterns of net error, of gross omission, and of misreporting of demographic characteristics are considerably more prevalent for the black population relative to the white. Fourth, the evidence suggests that considerable age misreporting exists in the official statistics. For example, for all four race-sex groups at ages 65-69 years, the estimates derived by demographic analysis suggest net *over*counts, whereas the Medicare linkage study found gross *omissions* in the magnitude of 2.1% (for white, females) to 12.6% (for black and other races, males). This implies that while these groups have gross omissions in the number of persons enumerated at ages 65-69, other larger errors (i.e., age misreporting) are operating in the other direction to cause a net overcount at these ages. The Medicare evaluation study of age misreporting, while problematic because individuals aged under 65 in Medicare were not included in the sample population, suggests that this interpretation is valid. A consequence of the pattern of gross error into the aged category is that the characteristics of a substantial part of the population reported as 65 and over in the Census relate in fact to persons under 65 (US Bureau of the Census, 1976).

The Census Bureau (1976), however, notes: "In spite of the limitations, it is believed that the general magnitudes, relations, and patterns are reflected satisfactorily by the reported figures, except perhaps at the very extreme ages. In any case, small differentials should be disregarded or at least viewed with caution."

EVALUATION OF THE 1980 CENSUS

Official tabulations of the 1980 population are presented in *Series B--US Summary of the 1980 Census* (US Bureau of the Census, 1983a). As was the case with the official 1970 Census statistics, these tabulations are known to contain certain evident errors.

In the official 1980 census, a number of problems related to classification of race exist. First, a large number of Spanish-origin persons self-reported their race differently in the 1980 census than in the 1970 census; this difference in reporting has a substantial impact on the counts and comparability for the "white" and the "other race" populations. To be more specific, a much larger proportion of the Spanish-origin population in 1980 than in 1970 reported their race as "other race."

Second, the Census Bureau made modifications in the treatment of certain persons of Hispanic and/or Asian Indian classification. As was the case in the 1970 census, the "white" category included those persons who self-reported their race as white, as well as persons who did not classify themselves in one of the specific race categories listed on the questionnaire but entered a response such as Polish, European, or Lebanese. The "black" category contained individuals who self-reported their race as "black" plus those who wrote in a response such as Jamaican, black Puerto Rican, West Indian, or Nigerian. The modification involved persons who did not classify themselves in one of the specific race categories but marked "other" and wrote in Hispanic entries such as Cuban, Puerto Rican, Mexican, or Dominican. In the 1970 census, these persons were reclassified as "white." In the 1980 census, however, most of these persons remained in the "other races" category.

As a result of this procedural change and the differences in reporting by this population, the proportion of the Spanish-origin population classified as "other race" in the 1980 census was substantially higher than that in the 1970 census. Nationally, in 1970, only one percent of the Spanish-origin persons were classified as "other" race; 93% were reported as "white." In 1980, a much larger proportion, 40%, of Spanish-origin persons reported their race as "other" and only 56% reported "white."

A third race-related problem related to the classification of Asian Indians. In 1980, the category "Asian Indian" was added as a separate response category to the race question. In the 1980 census, individuals (N=362,000) who chose this response were included in the "other races" category. In contrast, in the 1970 census, these individuals (N=100,000) were classified as "white."

As a consequence of these differences, originally published 1980 population totals for "white" and "other" are not comparable with corresponding 1970 figures, nor are they analogous to other data sources (birth and death registration, Medicare, net immigration statistics, Social Security administrative records, etc). To conform to historical categories of the racial groupings, the Census Bureau redistributed the 1980 census data. This modification of the racial data in the 1980 census added 6.3 million persons, or 3.4%, to the white category and 188,000 persons, or 0.7%, to the black population. The "other races" category decreased by 6.5 million (55.9% of the originally tabulated population of the "other" category) (US Bureau of the Census, 1988). In the population aged 60 and above, the modifications added 140,608 white males (an increase of 1.04%), 173,978 white females (0.93%), 3,979 black males (0.32%), and 6,133 black females (0.35%).

A final race-related complication involved allocation of the characteristic for persons of mixed parentage who did not select one of the designated races. In the 1970 census, such persons were allocated to the race of the father. In the 1980 census, however, assignment was made to the race of the mother.

Aside from race-related issues, other errors are known to exist in the 1980 official tabulations. Independent estimates of the number of persons aged 100 and over indicate that the number of centenarians enumerated in the 1980 census has been overstated, but to a much lesser degree than in the 1970 enumeration. For comparison, the 1980 census enumerated 32,194 persons aged 100 and above, whereas Social Security roles carry approximately 15,000 individuals of the same age (US Bureau of the Census, 1984a).

Evaluations of the accuracy of the 1980 census were also undertaken to determine the amount and sources of net error (see US Bureau of the Census, 1988). The studies were based on both demographic analysis and the 1980 Post Enumeration Program (PEP). The next section provides a detailed description of the undercount estimates based on demographic analysis. That is followed by estimates obtained from the PEP program. Finally, a section which presents a summarizing evaluation of the quality of the old-age population statistics in the 1980 census is provided.

Evaluation of 1980 Census using Demographic Analysis

For the demographic analysis, the Census Bureau used aggregate Medicare enrollments which were adjusted for under-enrollment to estimate the population aged 65 and above. Revisions of estimates of total white births initially derived by Whelpton for 1915-1935 (National Office of Vital Statistics, 1950) were utilized by Census to estimate the white population aged 45-64 in 1980. Expected sex ratios were used to derive the black, male population aged 45-64 in 1980, whereas Coale-Rives (1973) estimates were used for the black, female population of the same age.

As before, the method of demographic analysis relied upon independent aggregate data sources such as births, deaths, immigration, Medicare enrollments, expected sex ratios, etc. to estimate the total US population and its components by race, sex, and age group. An increasingly important limitation of the method over time is its required adjustment for the incompleteness of any of the component data. The census undercount estimates have generally been highly robust to the adjustment assumptions of the independent data sources. In the years prior to the 1980 census, however, the magnitude of the undocumented immigrant population resident in the United States gained in importance relative to the magnitude of the census undercount. Yet, no method independent of the 1980 census has provided reliable estimates of that population (US Bureau of the Census, 1988). Hence, the Census Bureau varied its estimates of undocumented aliens in the range of 2.0 to 5.0 million to derive various estimates of the net error rates by demographic analysis. The impact of the varying estimates of the undocumented population on the coverage estimates has been modest for the aged population for two reasons. First, the highest immigration rates are observed in young adulthood. Second, the relative importance of mortality as a component of change far outweighs the contribution of net undocumented immigration.

Table 2.8 presents estimates of net census error in the 1980 census derived by demographic analysis. Net overcounts are evident for all race-sex groups at ages 65-69 and ages 70-74. White females also exhibit an overcount for age group 60-64. This pattern suggests possible age misreporting into the age groups with net overcounts, particularly from age group 60-64 (except for white females).

Table 2.8

Preferred Estimates of Net Underenumeration, in Absolute Numbers and Percent: 1980 Census, by Sex, Race, and Age

	Undercount (in Thousands)			
	Whites		Blacks	
Age	Males	Females	Males	Females
All Ages	1,181	-222	1,169	409
55-59 years	122	-44	56	9
60-64 years	79	-18	27	1
65-69 years	-6	-62	-10	-28
70-74 years	-2	-9	-4	-8
75 years & over	36	167	2	31
65 years & over	28	96	-12	-5

Table 2.8 (continued)

Net Underenumeration (in Percent)

Age	Whites Males	Whites Females	Blacks Males	Blacks Females	Difference Blacks-Whites Males	Difference Blacks-Whites Females
Total	1.2	-0.2	8.5	2.8	7.3	3.0
55-59	2.4	-0.8	10.7	1.6	8.3	2.4
60-64	1.8	-0.4	6.6	0.2	4.8	0.6
65-69	-0.2	-1.4	-3.0	-6.8	2.8	5.4
70-74	-0.1	-0.3	-1.9	-2.5	1.8	2.2
75+	1.1	2.8	0.6	6.3	0.5	3.5
65+	0.3	0.7	-1.2	-0.4	1.5	1.1

Notes: (1) Estimates have been adjusted for reclassification by race, as discussed in the text, (2) All figures rounded independently, (3) Estimates include about 38,000 undocumented immigrants who were enumerated in the 1980 census; (4) A minus sign denotes a net overcount.

Source: US Bureau of the Census, 1988. Extracted from Appendix A.80.2.

Comparing the net census error rates of blacks and whites, the black errors are generally larger than that of whites. The overcount rate (6.8%) for black females aged 65 to 69, for instance, is almost five times the over-enumeration for white females of the same age (1.4%).

Contrasting sexes, the female net error rates are generally larger than that of the males in these aged categories, except at ages 60-64. This contrasts with estimates for the population of all ages, in which error rates for males exceed those of females. The differences between sexes are generally smaller, however, than that experienced by the racial groupings. The rates in 1980 are often lower than the comparable values in 1970.

Evaluation of the 1980 Census by Record Matching

The demographic methods provided estimates of the net census error, but do not yield measurements of its component parts. To that end, the 1980 Post Enumeration Program (PEP) employed record matching and sample survey methods for a sample of persons to estimate omissions and erroneous inclusions in the census. The PEP consisted of three separate surveys. The first two, referred to as the "P" or "population" samples, contained: (1) the April 1980 sample of the CPS, encompassing approximately 84,000 households, (2) the August sample of the CPS, which was of the same estimated size, and a military supplement since the CPS samples interviewed only the civilian, non-institutionalized population. Note that a separate P sample of the institutionalized population was also conducted but its results are not incorporated into the national estimates. The purpose of the P samples was to evaluate gross omissions from the census by matching samples of persons against the census enumerations. The third survey is referred to as the "E" or "enumeration" sample. It consists of approximately 110,000 households sampled from the 1980 census itself. The objective of the E sample was to determine to what extent persons were duplicated or individuals were wrongfully included in the census (US Bureau of the Census, 1988).

For the Post-Enumeration Program (PEP) match study, 29 alternative estimates of the coverage of the population in the 1980 census were created, reflecting the uncertainty of the underlying assumptions that had to be made to produce the estimates (US Bureau of the Census, ibid). For simplification, presentation of results will be limited to 4 alternative sets of estimates, representing the range of all values.

As evidenced by Table 2.9, the PEP estimates vary widely and differ significantly from the estimates obtained by demographic analysis in most cases. In each age-sex combination considered for the black population, the PEP range overlapped both negative and positive values, indicating that even the direction (overcount or undercount) is indeterminate. Furthermore, for both racial categories, in a majority of cases, the estimates obtained from demographic analysis are outside the range of PEP estimates. The dissimilarities between the demographic and PEP estimates are most evident for blacks. In only

Quality of the Decennial Census Data on the Older Population 45

one case, that of black females aged 60-64, does the demographic estimate (0.2%) fall within the range of PEP estimates (-1.0 to +2.1%), and even then there is uncertainty about the direction of error.

Estimates obtained from demographic analysis exhibited higher error rates for females (relative to males) for both races in all age categories aged 65 and above. Nonetheless, the PEP failed to confirm differential undercount rates by sex. The Census Bureau (1988) notes, however, that the estimates from demographic analysis are so strong and internally consistent that its results are judged as more accurate. Butz (1991) further notes that high rates of missing data in the post-enumeration program in 1980 contributed to the uncertainty in coverage estimates.

The Census Bureau summarizes that "the degree of agreement between the demographic analysis and PEP estimates for the total population or a racial group in any of the PEP sets is in large part a fortuitous circumstance." (US Bureau of the Census, 1988). Nonetheless, detailed analysis of the PEP results contributed two important conclusions for the understanding of the nature of census error in 1980. First, "the PEP confirmed results from the 1980 Housing Unit Enumeration Duplication Study that an appreciable fraction of the total census count, probably in excess of 1.1 percent, represented duplicate enumerations of persons already in the census. Although equally thorough evaluations of duplications had not been conducted for earlier censuses, the evidence implies much lower levels of duplication then. Thus, regrettably, duplication receives dubious credit for part of the improvement in 1980 in net census coverage." (US Bureau of the Census, 1988). Second, the PEP verified that gross errors in the census (incorrect omissions and duplicate enumerations) are larger than the estimated net error. This is a result of the cancelling effects of the two sources of error.

Table 2.9

Estimates of Net Undercount in the 1980 Census, as Derived by Demographic Analysis and by Alternative Post-Enumeration Program Estimates

Race and Age	DEM	PEP 3-8	PEP 5-8	PEP 10-8	PEP 14-8	PEP RANGE
Black Males						
60-64 years	6.6	1.6	0.4	-0.4	-1.0	-0.4 to 3.8
65-69 years	-3.0	2.0	3.2	2.2	-0.5	-0.4 to 3.8
70-74 years	-1.9	1.9	3.2	2.2	-0.5	-0.5 to 4.2
75 years and over	0.6	-2.6	-1.7	-2.7	-5.0	-5.0 to 0.5
Black Females						
60-64 years	0.2	1.4	-0.7	-1.0	-0.4	-1.0 to 2.1
65-69 years	-6.8	0.2	1.3	0.9	-1.5	-1.5 to 2.3
70-74 years	-2.5	0.0	1.1	0.7	-1.6	-1.6 to 2.1
75 years and over	6.3	-0.9	0.9	0.5	-1.9	-1.9 to 1.8

Table 2.9 (continued)

Race and Age	DEM	PEP 3-8	PEP 5-8	PEP 10-8	PEP 14-8	PEP RANGE
White & Other Males						
60-64 years	1.7	-0.5	-0.4	-0.8	-1.4	-1.4 to -0.1
65-69 years	-0.3	-1.2	-1.0	-1.2	-1.7	-1.7 to -0.7
70-74 years	-0.2	-1.3	-1.1	-1.5	-1.9	-1.9 to -0.7
75 years and over	0.9	-1.9	-1.5	-1.9	-2.5	-2.5 to -1.1
White & Other Females						
60-64 years	-0.5	-1.9	-1.4	-1.6	-2.6	-2.6 to -1.2
65-69 years	-1.5	-1.4	-1.5	-1.7	-2.0	-2.0 to -0.8
70-74 years	-0.3	-1.0	-1.7	-1.9	-1.7	-1.9 to -0.7
75 years and over	2.6	-0.2	-1.4	-1.7	-1.5	-1.7 to 0.1

Notes: (1) Demographic estimates include an allowance for 2.06 million undocumented residents counted in the 1980 census, (2) - signifies a net overcount, (3) All figures rounded independently, (4) Base of percent is the estimated population, (5) Estimates are compared to census counts classified by modified race, (6) PEP: Post-Enumeration Program: described in text.

Source: US Bureau of the Census, 1988.

Summary Evaluation: Quality of Old-Age Population Statistics in the 1980 Census

In spite of the inconsistencies between the two sets of estimates, a number of conclusions can be inferred concerning the completeness of the 1980 census. First, the magnitude of net error in the old-age statistics is greater than for the younger population. Second, relative to the 1970 census, the net error rates in most of the aged race-sex groups were appreciably lower in 1980. However, results from the PEP and from the 1980 Housing Unit Enumeration Duplication Study affirm that a considerable proportion of the total census count, likely in excess of 1.1%, represented duplicate enumerations of individuals. Third, improvement in the coverage of the population was noted for both the black and the white populations. But, patterns of net error continue to be considerably more prevalent for the black population relative to the white. Fourth, demographic analysis convincingly suggests that differential error rates exist by sex in the aged categories, with females responses subject to a higher degree of error. Fifth, the evidence suggests that considerable age misreporting exists in the official statistics.

In summary, the pattern of errors in the 1980 census is similar to those in the 1970 census, differing mainly in magnitude. Two major differences, however, distinguish the 1980 census from its historical predecessors. First, for the first time ever, a significant number (an estimated 2.06 million) of undocumented residents were enumerated. And, second, a considerably higher level of duplication of individuals is noted for the 1980 census.

EVALUATION OF THE 1990 CENSUS

Following historical precedent, the Census Bureau relied upon two primary methods to evaluate the undercount in the 1990 census. *Demographic analysis* used the demographic accounting equation (see equation 2.1) to reconstruct the population based on earlier censuses combined with data on vital events (births, deaths, and net immigration). In attempts to estimate the "true" population, the Census Bureau also attempted to match individuals enumerated in the *Post Enumeration Survey* (PES) to individuals enumerated in the census. Data on Medicare enrollment were also used to estimate the size of the population over the age of 65 (Schenker, 1993).

Modification of the official enumerations was again required to conform to historical data and administrative records. Two specific problems were identified in the evaluations of the quality of the 1990 census. The first difficulty involves inconsistencies in the reporting of race. The second entails misreporting of age by a single year due to misinterpretation of the Census question by about 10% of the respondents (US Bureau of the Census, 1991). The age issue is most pronounced at exact age 0.

Regarding race, in the 1990 enumerated census, 9.8 million persons (representing 3.9% of the total population count) wrote-in responses to the race question, as opposed to choosing one of the fifteen stipulated categories. About 95% of these cases were persons of Hispanic origin who reported their race as Mexican, Puerto Rican, etc. (Hollmann and Spencer, 1992a). For comparison, in 1980, a similar problem involved 6.3 million persons, representing 2.6% of the enumerated total population. Misunderstanding of the census age question was also identified as a potential source of error. First, individuals tended to report their ages as of the date of completion of the questionnaire, rather than as of April 1st, the requested date. Second, persons who approached their birthday tended to round up their age (US Bureau of the Census, 1991). Hollmann and Spencer (1992a) estimate that about 10% of persons in most single year of age categories are actually one year younger, but the misstatements are largely offsetting, with relatively equal numbers of persons reporting into and out of an age category. At exact age 0, however, a large discrepancy exists, because age misreporting was uni-directional upward. No one moves up to age 0.

Published data from the 1990 census does not correct for either the detailed race or age problems. Instead, adjustments of the enumerated data, made on an individual record basis, were incorporated into what has come to be referred to as the MARS (*M*odified *A*ge and *R*ace *S*tatistics) file. The modified file allows comparison of the 1990 census data with historical censuses and other forms of demographic data (death and birth records, Medicare enrollments, etc.). For specifics of the modification methodology, see Hollmann and Spencer (1992a) and Robinson et al. (1991).

It should be noted that the modified file adjusts only for the two specified race and age problems. No modification was made for other important sources of error. Continuing problems in the age data include age misreporting, heaping on year of birth, and inaccuracies in the statistics of the oldest old. Similarly, other problems related to the race characteristic continue to exist. These include changes in census coverage over time, and, variations in the respondents' self-identification with a racial group over time (which results in differential race reporting in censuses over time and in administrative records for the same individual). Furthermore, the MARS file simultaneously corrects for both the age and the race problems. Decomposed estimates of error by cause are not available.

Evaluation of 1990 Census using Demographic Analysis

The general method of demographic analysis as a tool for coverage evaluation has been actively used at the US Bureau of the Census to assess the completeness of coverage in every census since 1960 (Robinson et al., 1993). Table 2.10 presents estimates derived by demographic analysis of the amount and percent of net undercount in the 1990 census by age, sex, and race.

Over the four decade period from 1940 to 1980, the percent undercount of the overall population decreased steadily from about 5.4% in 1940 to about 1.2% in 1980. Between 1980 and 1990, however, a reversal was noted. Census coverage in 1990, estimated to measure about 1.85% (or 4.7 million persons) was worse relative to 1980 (Robinson et al, *ibid*; Schenker, *ibid*). It has been speculated that this result may have been due to the high degree of duplications in the 1980 census, rather than to a worsening of census coverage in 1990.

Based Table 2.10, a number of generalizations can be made regarding the pattern of net undercount in the 1990 census for the aged population. First, following its historical trend, the net error estimates for blacks surpass those of nonwhites by a wide margin. The largest differential is noted for males aged 60-64. The net undercount rate for blacks equals 10.3 percent, surpassing the white estimate of 2.6 percent by 7.7 percentage points. Second, while at most ages net error rates for males surpass those of female, a number of notable exceptions occur in the aged statistics. In the statistics for blacks, female net error rates are in excess at ages 65-69 and ages 75 and above. For nonblacks, female error rates surpass male rates only at ages 75 and above. Third, whereas undercounts are observed for all of the male aged categories, overcounts are noted in many of the female age groups. Fourth, as noted by Robinson et al (1992), the net coverage patterns are generally consistent across the last three censuses for each race-sex group.

Table 2.10

Estimates of Amount and Percent of Net Undercount in the 1990 Census, Derived by Demographic Analysis, by Age, Sex, and Race

	Blacks				Non-Blacks			
	Males		Females		Males		Females	
Age	Amt	%	Amt	%	Amt	%	Amt	%
All	1,338	8.5	498	3.0	2,142	2.0	706	0.6
55-59	63	12.1	0	0.0	140	3.0	17	0.4
60-64	48	10.3	-15	-2.9	120	2.6	4	0.1
65-69	8	2.1	-36	-7.7	95	2.2	-48	-0.9
70-74	11	4.1	-14	-3.8	60	1.9	-4	-0.1
75+	11	3.2	30	4.4	7	0.2	120	1.5

Source: Robinson, J.B., B. Ahmed, P.D Gupta, and K.A. Woodrow. 1993. Estimation of population coverage in the 1990 United States census based on demographic analysis. *Journal of the American Statistical Association, Special Section on Undercount in 1990 Census.* Vol. 88, No. 423, pp. 1061-1071.

Clifford and Himes (1993), while endorsing demographic analysis as a method for providing useful information about undercount rates and trends, note however that a significant number of demographic analysis evaluation projects had to be carried out by the Census Bureau in order to capture the sources and magnitude of uncertainty in the components of population change. Because the final output produced by the Census Bureau, i.e. interval estimates for undercount rates, is determined primarily by these assumptions, they recommend that it would be valuable: (1) to determine just how variable expert judgments on bounds for the particular components are, (2) to recognize that the spirit of the operation is Bayesian (not frequentist), and (3) to derive empirical or sampling-based expressions for plausible distributions of particular components.

Evaluation of the 1990 Census Based on the PES

The 1990 Post Enumeration Survey (PES) consisted of two parts. The first part was a sample of the population, known as the *P* sample. The proportion of the *P* sample included in the census is an estimate of the proportion of the total population included in the census. The second part, the *E* sample, consisted of a sample of the census enumerations used to estimate the proportion of erroneous enumerations. These enumerations were checked against the census itself to determine the extent of duplication (Hogan, 1993). The population was divided into post-strata based on geography, race, origin, housing tenure, age, and sex.

Table 2.11

Undercounts in the 1990 Census Estimates Based on Comparison of the Census with the Post Enumeration Survey (PES)

Population Sub-Group	Undercount Estimate (in percent)
Overall, Total	1.6
Non-Hispanic White & Other	0.7
Black	4.6
Hispanic	5.0
Asian & Pacific Islander	2.4
Reservation Indian	12.2

Source: Hogan, 1993.

The census estimates showed a net national undercount of 2.1%, later adjusted to 1.6%. Higher undercount rates were measured for blacks as well as for Hispanics and Asians when compared to whites (see Table 2.11). Had the census been adjusted based on the final PES results, the official count of the resident population would have increased by almost 4.0 million persons. There are *net* numbers. In reality, 5.45 million records would have been added to account for net undercount, and 1.46 million records subtracted to account for net overcount (Hogan, *ibid*).

While Hogan (1993) also calculated estimates by age and sex, these results were not presented.

Summary Evaluation: Quality of Population Statistics in the 1990 Census

While the specific results from the demographic analysis studies and those of the post enumeration survey are in conflict, major conclusions are clear. In contrast to the 1940-1980 period, when net undercount rates were continually declining over time, by 1990, net undercount not only failed to improve, but appears to have gotten appreciably worse. As noted by Passel (1993), the black-white differential in coverage got larger, and in fact may be as great as it has ever been (at least in the 1940-1990 period for which we have consistent measures). Robinson et al. (1993) suggest that improvements in the 1990 census operations led to fewer duplications than in 1980, with a resulting increase in net undercount rates.

AGE HEAPING AND RACIAL MISCLASSIFICATION

Two final data quality issues will be considered in the evaluation of US census data in 1970, 1980, and 1990: the degree of age heaping and racial misclassification.

Age Heaping

Age heaping is defined by Pressat (1988) as a general tendency to misreport a preferred number as one's age (for example a number thought to be lucky, such as seven, or honorable, such as 100) or to round one's age to a number ending with the digits zero or five. Based on Myers' summary index of age misreporting, age heaping was diminished to such low levels in the 1970 and 1980 censuses that it could not readily be differentiated from other errors in the data and from real fluctuations due to past variations in births, deaths, and net migration (US Bureau of the Census, 1983a). For 1990, however, there appears to be slight heaping on "year of birth" for years ending in 0 and 5.

Race Misclassification

The discussion of data quality in the censuses has largely focused on issues of census completeness and quality of age reporting. While it is certainly recognized that inconsistencies in the reporting of race can introduce appreciable errors into the data sources, only limited information is available about differences in reporting of race among the various sources or over time.

Two sources of inconsistency in race classification exist: (1) categorization of children of mixed race parents, and, (2) variations in the reporting of race by adults over time, particularly for the black race group (Robinson and Lapham, 1991). The latter could be expected to have a larger impact at the older ages.

The limited empirical evidence suggests that black adults have not significantly changed their racial identification over time. Robinson and Lapham (1991) cite evidence from two sources: match studies and external evidence. They note that match studies (see US Bureau of the Census, 1973, 1975; McKenney, Fernandez, and Masumura, 1980) conducted in conjunction with the 1970 and 1980 censuses found that the black population in the census was about one percent lower than the interview-based population. An opposing result was found, however, in a matching study of the 1970 census with Medicare records for the population aged 65 and over. The black-and-other races population in the census was four percent larger in the census than in Medicare. While the result was found to be statistically significant, the interpretation should be viewed with caution for a number of reasons. First, the match study used originally-published census statistics although a number of improvements in racial classification (particularly for the Hispanic population) were incorporated into a later modified file. Second, the results were not presented separately for blacks. While blacks generally constitute about 90% of the nonwhite category, significant misreporting of race in the other racial categories could bias the result. Various diverse studies support the contention that nonwhites (other than blacks) have much higher rates of race misreporting. Passel and Berman (1986) have presented evidence of significant misreporting of race into the American Indian category in the 1980 census. The 1980 census enumeration of American Indians, Eskimos, and Aleuts was more than 70 percent higher than the corresponding 1970 census count. Poe (1992) reports significantly higher differences in the reporting of race between the death certificate and the 1986 National Mortality Followback Survey for members of the "other race" category. In a study in which infant death certificates were matched to birth records, a different race was reported in 31.2 percent of the Native American cases, 8.4 percent of the Asian, 3.0 percent of white non-Hispanic, and only 1.7 percent for African Americans (Farley, Richards, and Bell, no date). Finally, the number of matched cases for males of the black and other races category in the Census-Medicare study was only 972. Four percent misreporting of race would require only 39 individuals to report differently on both sources.

Robinson and Lapham (1991) also present external evidence to support the contention that blacks have not changed their racial self-identification in large numbers. First, Coale-Rives estimates of coverage for the black population (Coale and Rives, 1973), which are based on the reconstruction of a long historical series of census data from 1880 to 1970, exhibit a high degree of internal consistency. Second, estimates of net coverage for 1970 and 1980 based on Medicare or Social Security are internally consistent. Finally, the examination of error of closure measures by race and sex for the censuses between 1950 and 1980 does not reveal the presence of major inconsistencies in the reporting of race.

III

Evaluation of the Death Registration and Immigration Statistics

Population change for the aged between two censuses can only occur through two main mechanisms: through death or through net immigration. This chapter provides a detailed review of evaluations of the US death registration data, as well as statistics on immigration and emigration.

DEATH REGISTRATION DATA

Official death statistics, published by the National Center for Health Statistics (NCHS), are the basic source of annual mortality data in the United States. The figures are generally utilized without adjustment for underregistration or for misreporting of characteristics on the death certificate. It is generally assumed that the death registration system is practically complete (Wilkin, 1981; US Bureau of the Census, 1984a; NCHS, 1968) although no national test of its comprehensiveness has been conducted since the completion of the Death Registration Area in 1933 (Preston et al, 1991). This assumption is based on the strict legal requirements for registration as well of the needs of survivors for proof of death in connection with burial, settling estates and collecting insurance benefits (US Bureau of the Census, 1984; Wilkin, 1981). Calculations by Coale and Kisker (1990), however, suggest that underregistration of deaths exists, particularly at the older ages. For the nonwhite population, for instance, registered deaths were 7% fewer than Medicare deaths for the male population aged over age 80 in 1980, whereas registered female deaths were 10%

fewer. These numbers, however, may be reflective of differential age reporting between the two sources, rather than underenumeration.

A second serious problem affecting the use of official death statistics is the misreporting of demographic characteristics of the decedents on the death certificate. The quality of some attributes has been widely studied including "cause of death" and "occupation and industry" (see Poe et al, 1992 for an exhaustive listing of citations). Evaluations of the quality of data on age, race, and sex, however, have been sparse, particularly for the 1970 to 1990 time frame.

The following sections provide summaries of recent investigations of the quality of death registration data.

Linkage of Death Certificates to the 1986 National Mortality Followback Survey

An evaluation of reporting of demographic items on the death certificate was recently undertaken at the National Center for Health Statistics (NCHS) by Poe et al (1992). In this study, the authors linked death certificates selected from the 1986 Current Mortality Sample (CMS) to responses on the 1986 National Mortality Followback Survey (NMFS), a nationally representative (except Oregon) sample that questioned the death certificate informant (generally the next of kin) within one year following the death of an adult in 1986. The CMS is a ten-percent sample of death certificates received by the state vital statistics offices and transmitted to the NCHS. The NMFS is a sample conducted by NCHS to gauge the reliability of demographic items reported on the death certificate of adults aged 25 and older.

Based on information for 18,733 decedents, there was only 77.5% agreement between exact age as reported on the death certificate and exact age as reported on the followback questionnaire for the total population. Table 3.1 presents the percent exact age agreement between the two data sources at the older ages.

In general, the degree of exact agreement between the two sources decreased as the age of the decedent increased. The lowest agreement (78.7%) for whites was found in age group 70-79; and for blacks in age group 80-89 (62.4%). Agreement on the race variable was found to be excellent, as seen in Table 3.2. For whites in each of the old-age categories, percent agreement was found to be greater than or equal to 98.6%; for blacks greater than or equal to 97.0%.

Table 3.1

Age of Decedent: Percent of Cases from the 1986 National Mortality Followback Survey in Exact Agreement with the Death Certificate, by Race

Race on Death Certificate	Age of Decedent on Death Certificate				
	All Ages	60-69	70-79	80-89	90+
All Races	77.5	77.2	74.0	75.4	78.2
Whites	81.6	83.4	78.7	79.2	82.1
Blacks	67.1	66.5	62.5	62.4	64.9

Source: Poe, G. et al., 1992. Comparability of reporting of demographic items between the death certificate and the 1986 National Mortality Followback Survey. Draft dated 5/14/92. Table B.

Table 3.2

Race of Decedent: Percent of Cases from the 1986 National Mortality Followback Survey in Exact Agreement with the Death Certificate, by Age

Age on Death Certificate	Race of Decedent on Death Certificate		
	All Races	Whites	Blacks
All Ages	97.9	98.2	98.0
60-69	98.3	98.6	98.2
70-79	98.3	98.7	98.1
80-89	98.5	98.8	98.4
90 and over	98.3	98.8	97.0

Source: Poe, G. et al., 1992. Comparability of reporting of demographic items between the death certificate and the 1986 National Mortality Followback Survey. Draft dated 5/14/92. Table B.

Table 3.3

Comparability of Age of Decedent as Reported on Death Certificate and the NMFS for Population Aged 60 & Above, by Time Interval between Death and the Survey
(Percent of Cases)

Interval (in weeks)	Number	Age at Death on NMFS Questionnaire Compared to Death Certificate Age		
		Younger	Same	Older
22-25	730	1.8	94.8	3.4
26-29	1447	1.5	95.2	3.3
30-32	1270	1.3	95.4	3.3
33-35	1530	2.2	93.2	4.6
36-38	1300	3.0	92.0	5.0
39-41	1094	3.9	91.1	4.9
42-44	972	4.8	89.0	6.2
45-47	657	4.1	89.2	6.7
48-51	496	5.6	88.7	5.6
52+	455	4.2	88.8	7.0
Missing	9	11.1	88.9	0.0

Notes: (1) NMFS: National Mortality Followback Survey; (2) Comparability between sources is evaluated within 5-year age groups (open-ended at age 95), so the % of cases in agreement overstates "exact" agreement; (3) The average interval between death and the NMFS for decedents aged 60 and above was 36.6 weeks as calculated from grouped data. We made two adjustments to the data: (a) cases in which the interval data was missing were dropped; and, (b) mid-point of open-ended interval was assumed to be 60 weeks.

Source: Poe, G. et al., 1992. Comparability of reporting of demographic items between the death certificate and the 1986 National Mortality Followback Survey. Draft dated 5/14/92. Detailed Tables: Table 1.

A limitation of the study is its inability to ascertain which of the data sources, if any, had the correct age. A further limitation was that it failed to control for the interval between the death and the followback survey, although a strong relationship between percent agreeing on exact age in number of years and the interval between the death and survey was noted. Although the age at death should be the same on both the death certificate and in the followback survey, as shown in Table 3.3, the probability of a misreported age by followback survey respondents increased as the interval since death increased.

Linkage of the National Longitudinal Mortality Study with the National Death Index

In another recent study, Sorlie et al (1992) evaluated the validity of race and sex characteristics on the death certificate in a linkage study. Using the National Longitudinal Mortality Study, the authors identified 43,520 deaths for which distinguishing data were available on both the CPS and the National Death Index. Overall, the authors found high percentage agreement between characteristics on the CPS and characteristics on the death certificate. For race, the percentage agreement was 99.4%, overall. For whites, 99.2%; for blacks, 98.2%. Percent agreement for the sex characteristic was also high, at 99.5%. Although detailed results were not presented, the authors note that the rates of agreement do not vary considerably by sex/age group of the decedent. Limitations of the study were its failure to evaluate the validity of age characteristics on the death certificate and characteristics of persons with missing data.

Linkage of Death Certificates to Improved Social Security/Medicare Administrative Records

Another recent study involved the linkage of death certificates in two states (Texas and Massachusetts) to improved social security/Medicare administrative records for the elderly population (Kestenbaum, 1990; no date). The results of this study are summarized in Table 3.4.

Table 3.4

Percentage Agreement between the Death Certificate and Improved Medicare Enrollment Data

Characteristics	Ages 65 & Over		Ages 85 & Over	
	Same Exact Age	Same 5-Year Interval	Same Exact Age	Same 5-Year Interval
TOTAL, All Matched Records	92.5	97.2	89.4	96.2
RACE				
White, not Hispanic	94.6	98.2	91.7	97.2
Black	72.6	87.0	63.2	84.6
Hispanic	88.4	95.5	81.7	92.8
AGE				
65-69	95.4	98.1	----	----
70-74	94.6	97.9	----	----
75-79	93.6	97.4	----	----
80-84	92.1	97.1	----	----
85-89	90.6	96.7	90.6	96.7
90-94	89.3	96.8	89.3	96.8
95-99	86.5	93.8	86.5	93.8
100 and over	80.1	88.6	80.1	88.6
SEX				
Male	94.2	98.0	91.0	96.9
Female	91.0	96.5	88.7	95.9

Source: Kestenbaum, B., 1992. A description of the extreme aged population based on improved Medicare enrollment data. Demography. 29(4):565-580. Table 4.

Evaluation of Death Registration and Immigration Statistics   63

In general, Kestenbaum (1990) highlights very high rates of agreement on age. For the total population aged 65 and above, the percent agreement on exact age was found to be 92.5%. For ages 85 and above, the agreement fell to 89.4%. In five-year intervals, the percent agreement increased to 97.2% and 96.2%, respectively. Note however that the accord is greatly enhanced by high agreement for the "whites, not Hispanic" group. For the total black population aged 65 and above, exact age matched only 72.6% of the time, and for the black population aged 85 and above, this figure drops to 63.2%. In summary, Kestenbaum found: (1) lower percent agreement for old-age blacks, relative to non-Hispanic whites and to Hispanics, (2) slightly lower agreement for females than males, even after controlling for age, and, (3) decreasing agreement as age increases.

Matching of Death Certificates with Census Records

An earlier evaluation (National Center for Health Statistics, 1968; Hambright, 1969), sometimes referred to as the Chicago mortality study, matched a national sample of death certificates from May to August 1960 with the 1960 census records. Although the data evaluated was collected before the time frame considered for this project, the study's findings provide insight into the continuing pattern of biases present in the death statistics. The authors found: (1) for whites, there was fairly constant agreement between sources with increasing age. For nonwhites, however, there was less agreement, (2) in the event of disagreement, discrepancies for the white population were generally within one year. For nonwhites, however, the average difference was more than one year, particularly at ages 45 and above, and, (3) For whites (all ages) and nonwhites (aged less than 45 years), the age reported on the death certificate was, on average, older than that reported on the census. For nonwhites aged 45 and above, however, age reported on the death certificate was younger than on the census.

Evaluation of US data from which US death rates are calculated

In order to study the accuracy of old-age death rates in the US, Coale and Kisker (1990) evaluated three sources of data: (1) registered deaths in 1980, (2) the population enumerated in the 1980 census, and (3) both the number of deaths and the number of persons enrolled in the Medicare program as of 1980 (and adjacent years). All data are classified by single years of age, race (white and nonwhite), and sex. While inconsistencies were more pronounced among nonwhites than among whites, the results differ somewhat for two age groups differentiated by Coale and Kisker: (1) above age 90 or 95 and (2) age 70 to 85 or 90. For the former age group, Coale and Kisker (1990:29) state: "we have found conclusive evidence of overstatement of age above age 90 or 95 in the 1980 census, in deaths registered in 1980, and in the population and deaths recorded in Medicare data for 1980." Having highlighted inconsistencies in the US data sources by use of internal and external consistency checks, Coale and Kisker (1990:4) note that "when age is imprecisely reported, international experience and past experience in the United States indicate a tendency toward progressively greater exaggeration of age as age increases." By introducing a pattern of mild overstatement of age beginning at age 70, Coale and Kisker produced mortality rates for older whites which approximate those observed in other low-mortality European countries.

For age group 70 to 85 or 90, Coale and Kisker found less direct evidence but cited the possibility of overstatement of age in all three of the data sources. The possibility was implied by (1) an abnormally slow rate of increase in death rates above age 65 and a less steeply declining age distribution compared with other low mortality populations, and (2) the tendency to round ages or birthdays, as evidenced by age heaping (Coale and Kisker, ibid).

Coale and Kisker further suggest that underregistration of deaths exists at the older ages, particularly in the African American population. This conclusion is based on two observations. First, fewer registered deaths are recorded at older ages in the vital statistics than in Medicare records. Second, populations above age 80 reconstructed from deaths using variable-r procedures developed by Preston and Coale (1982) are too small relative to census counts in 1980. As noted earlier, however, these differences may be reflective of differential age reporting between the two sources rather than underenumeration.

While the analyses of Coale and Kisker certainly highlight inconsistencies between the census, the death registration system, and Medicare records in 1980, the procedures employed to attribute the errors are insufficient. Numerous different patterns and magnitudes of age misreporting and coverage error at the older ages could produce the same results. Even as noted by Coale and Kisker (1990:5), "the corrections for age overstatement . . . are somewhat arbitrary estimates. Different corrections of about the same magnitude would be equally well justified. Our tables . . . show the distorting effect of age overstatement on US mortality patterns at high ages, but the exact extent of distortion can only be guessed. Nevertheless, they are a sensible approximation of "true" mortality rates" at the oldest ages.

Matching of 1900 Census with Death Certificates

All of the cited studies highlight inconsistencies in the reporting of demographic characteristics between sources at a point in time. For the age characteristic, however, these analyses fail in two important aspects. First, they are unable to ascertain which data source, if either, provides the "true" age. Second, since most comparisons are done at points close in time, they fail to capture the degree to which characteristic reporting has changed over time by individuals in a cohort.

To minimize age exaggeration, one would need to link an individual's birth certificate with his death certificate. For persons born outside of (or before) the Birth Registration Area, linkage could be attempted with censuses conducted early in the life of the decedent. This methodology was employed by Rosenwaike and Logue (1983) in an innovative study designed to verify age reporting on the death certificate for the population aged 85 and over in the 1968 to 1972 period. The authors selected a sample of death records from those filed for decedents of extreme age in Pennsylvania and New Jersey. Linkage to the 1900 manuscript census of population was accomplished for a total of 1429 decedents, of which 960 were white and 469 were nonwhite. The original sample size was 1511 whites and 1666 blacks.

Referring to Tables 3.5 and 3.6, Rosenwaike and Logue found a number of interesting results. First, age agreement of matched census records with death certificates decreased as age increased for both racial groups. Second, striking differences were noted between racial groups. Agreement levels for whites were high, except at ages 100 and over. For nonwhites, however, significantly lower agreement was found. Third, the authors note that, within race there was little difference by sex in agreement on age. Finally, for whites after age 90 there was a greater tendency for the death certificate age to be older than age at death calculated from age in the 1900 census. Before age 90, age on the death certificate was more likely to be younger than the presumably more accurate age derived from the 1900 census.

Table 3.5
Age Agreement on Census Records Matched with Death Certificates, by Race and Sex: New Jersey & Pennsylvania, 1968-72

Death Certificate Age Relative to Census Age	Whites			Blacks		
	Total	Males	Female	Total	Male	Female
	Number					
Within 0-11 months	693	221	472	186	72	114
1 year younger	68	19	49	37	21	16
1 year older	106	30	76	61	27	34
2 to 4 years younger	22	4	18	40	13	27
2 to 4 years older	52	16	36	72	30	42
5 or more yrs younger	5	4	1	13	6	7
5 or more years older	14	3	11	60	27	33
TOTAL	960	297	663	469	196	273

Table 3.5 (continued)

Percentage Distribution

	Whites			Blacks		
	Total	Male	Female	Total	Male	Female
Within 0-11 months	72.2	74.4	71.2	39.7	36.7	41.8
1 year younger	7.1	6.4	7.4	7.9	10.7	5.9
1 year older	11.0	10.1	11.5	13.0	13.8	12.5
2 to 4 years younger	2.3	1.3	2.7	8.5	6.6	9.9
2 to 4 years older	5.4	5.4	5.4	15.4	15.3	15.4
5 or more yrs younger	0.5	1.3	0.2	2.8	3.1	2.6
5 or more years older	1.5	1.0	1.7	12.8	13.8	12.1
TOTAL	100.0	100.0	100.0	100.0	100.0	100.0

Source: Rosenwaike, I. and B. Logue, 1983. Accuracy of death certificate ages for the extreme aged. *Demography* 20(4). Table 3.

Table 3.6
Age Agreement of Census Records Matched with Death Certificates, by Race and Age: New Jersey and Pennsylvania, by Number, 1968-72

Death Certif. Age Relative to Census Age	Whites 85-89 Years	Whites 90-94 Years	Whites 95-99 Years	Whites 100+ Years	Blacks 85-89 Years	Blacks 90-94 Years	Blacks 95-99 Years	Blacks 100+ Years
< 1 year	209	198	180	106	74	47	54	11
1 year younger	23	21	16	8	21	13	2	1
1 year older	11	29	41	25	24	20	16	1
2-4 yrs younger	4	8	6	4	19	12	8	1
2-4 yrs older	4	12	15	21	19	21	24	8
5/5+ yrs younger	1	3	1	0	6	4	3	0
5/5+ yrs older	1	4	5	4	10	8	21	21
Total	253	275	264	168	173	125	128	43
Exact Agreement	209	198	180	106	74	47	54	11
D.C. age younger	28	32	23	12	46	29	13	2
D.C. age older	16	45	61	50	53	49	61	30

Evaluation of Death Registration and Immigration Statistics 69

Table 3.6 (continued)
Age Agreement of Census Records Matched with Death Certificates, by Race and Age: New Jersey and Pennsylvania, by % Distribution, 1968-72

Death Certif. Age Relative to Census Age	Age on Death Certificate								
	Whites					Blacks			
	85-89 Years	90-94 Years	95-99 Years	100+ Years	85-89 Years	90-94 Years	95-99 Years	100+ Years
< 1 year	82.6	72.0	68.2	63.1	42.8	37.6	42.2	25.6
1 year younger	9.1	7.6	6.1	4.8	12.1	10.4	1.6	2.3
1 year older	4.3	10.5	15.5	14.9	13.9	16.0	12.5	2.3
2-4 yrs older	1.6	2.9	2.3	2.4	11.0	9.6	6.3	2.3
2-4 yrs younger	1.6	4.4	5.7	12.5	11.0	16.8	18.8	18.6
5/5+ yrs younger	0.4	1.1	0.4	0.0	3.5	3.2	2.3	0.0
5/5+ yrs older	0.4	1.5	1.9	2.4	5.8	6.4	16.4	48.8
Total	100.0	100.0	100.0	100.0	100.0	100.0	100.0	100.0
Exact Agreement	82.6	72.0	68.2	63.1	42.8	37.6	42.2	25.6
D.C. age younger	11.1	11.6	8.7	7.1	26.6	23.2	10.2	4.7
D.C. age older	6.3	16.4	23.1	29.8	30.6	39.2	47.7	69.8

The Rosenwaike and Logue study, while providing the only estimate of reported ages at death relative to "true" ages, has limitations. First, the information is now dated. Since evaluation was based on deaths in the 1968 to 1972 period, any change in the age misreporting pattern over the past thirty years remains unmeasured. Second, the authors evaluated the accuracy of reported age at death for only the extreme old population (aged 85 and above). Third, the analysis was affected by small sample size, particularly for nonwhites at the oldest ages. Finally, the study may not have been nationally-representative.

In the most ambitious examination of its kind to date, researchers at the University of Pennsylvania (Preston et al, 1991) are assessing the quality of age misreporting for African-American decedents in the 1980s. The evaluation methodology is to match a nationally-representative sample of death certificates from aged decedents (aged 60 and above) to the individuals' 1900, 1910, or 1920 census records and to administrative records from the Social Security Administration. Birth certificates will also be matched to death certificates for a sample of persons born in Maryland.

THE IMMIGRATION STATISTICS

To conform to the definition of "total resident population" discussed early in this chapter, accurate information is required for eight categories of immigration statistics: (1) alien immigration, (2) refugees and parolees, (3) net arrivals of civilian citizens, (4) net Puerto Rican migration, (5) emigration of residents from the United States, (6) net movement of resident foreign students, (7) net movement of US armed forces, and (8) net undocumented immigration. Yet, the lack of accurate and timely information on immigration matters is widely noted (Panel on Immigration Statistics, 1985). A committee in the House (House Report 98-759, 1984, cited in Panel on Immigration Statistics, 1985) notes that "the INS [Immigration and Naturalization Service] has not devoted sufficient resources and attention to this problem and, to a great extent, has ignored the statistical needs of Congress, as well as, the research needs of demographers and other outside users."

The US Bureau of the Census, however, compiles and corrects a wide variety of information on the flow and stock of migrants due to its need for immigration data for current population estimation and projection. We will rely heavily on these unpublished tabulations, which are the only known series of net immigration statistics available for the US population which incorporate all eight of the components listed by age, sex, and race.

The following section will present a descriptive summary of the component immigration statistics, based largely on information provided by the US Bureau of the Census (1987a). The alien immigration segment is believed to be both one of the more accurate and one of the more important (in terms of magnitude) components in the total net immigration statistics. These numbers are based on published annual reports of the Immigration and Naturalization Service (INS), Department of Justice, which provides data by age and sex for aliens admitted for permanent residence to the United States (US Bureau of the Census, 1987a). Since race is not collected by INS, estimation of this variable was generated at the Census Bureau based on reported country of origin.

As defined by the Panel on Immigration Statistics (1985), refugees are those persons outside their country of nationality who fear prosecution if they return. Parolees are persons allowed to enter the country under emergency conditions. Data on refugees and parolees are provided to Census by the Office of Refugee Resettlement of the US Department of Health and Human Services.

The classification "net arrivals of civilian citizens" is based on reports from the Department of Defense and the Office of Personnel Management, which estimates the change in the number of civilian Federal employees overseas, their dependents, and dependents of the Armed Forces overseas. No adjustment is made for the net movement of civilian citizens not affiliated with the Federal Government.

"Net Puerto Rican migration" measures the net movement of individuals between Puerto Rico and the United States mainland. Calculation of the estimate is described by Passel and Robinson (1988) as follows. "Data on the US resident population of Puerto Rican birth form the basis of the estimates of net migration from Puerto Rico. Parallel calculations are made for the Puerto Rican resident population of US birth to account for the out-migration of US-born persons to Puerto Rico. The algebraic sum of the two estimates represents net migration from Puerto Rico to the United States.

Since emigration (of residents from the United States) statistics are not collected by any US government agency, the US Census Bureau estimates the category. The estimates are based on evidence from foreign government censuses, analysis of the foreign-born population counted in the US censuses, and historical experience which has shown that total annual emigration in the US typically averages about thirty percent of total annual immigration.

The categories "net movement of resident foreign students" and "net movement of US armed forces" are inconsequential for this study because of small numbers in the aged groups. The former, however, is based on estimates from the International Institute for Education. The latter has been estimated by the US Department of Defense.

An undocumented resident immigrant refers to "a noncitizen physically present in the United States who entered the country illegally and has not regularized his or her situation, or who has violated his or her terms of entry." (Hill, 1985). Under the definition presented for resident population, these persons should be included in US population counts. Although the number present in the US has been the subject of extensive conjecture and study, no reliable estimates exist. Hill (ibid) summarized the findings of major studies (Goldberg, 1974; Lancaster and Scheuren, 1978; Robinson, 1980; Heer, 1979; Garcia y Griego, 1980; CENIET, 1982; Warren and Passel, 1983; Bean, King, and Passel, 1983) which evaluated the size of the illegal population, or components thereof, since the early 1970s. His review concludes that: (1) variations from method to method are large, (2) the estimates do not show a clear trend over time, (3) for those studies that produced estimates of upper and lower population limits, the range between the limits is typically large, (4) the procedures used all invoke assumptions that often cannot be adequately justified and to which the estimates obtained are sensitive, and, (5) the commonly quoted range of 3-6 million illegals may be too high.

IV

Adjustments to the Data Sources

The previous chapters focused on issues of completeness of coverage and misreporting of demographic characteristics for the older population in official data sources in the United States. Evaluation of three decennial censuses (1970, 1980, and 1990), the death registration, and net immigration statistics was provided.

The three censuses were evaluated by the US Bureau of the Census using various techniques, including demographic analysis, matching with administrative (Medicare) records, and matching with Current Population Survey (CPS) records. Based on these evaluation studies, a number of general conclusions were inferred regarding the quality of old-age population data in the censuses. Specifically:

1. The magnitude of net error in the old-age statistics is greater than for the younger population.

2. Patterns of net error, of gross omission, and of misreporting of demographic characteristics are considerably more prevalent for the African-American population relative to the white.

3. The evidence suggests that considerable age misreporting occurs in the data sources.

4. Age-specific net coverage patterns are generally consistent across the last three censuses for each race-sex group.

Differences do occur among the three censuses. The net error rates in most aged race-sex groups were appreciably lower in 1980 relative to 1970. While the improvement in coverage is discerned in both the African American and the white populations, net error is still more prevalent for African Americans. Results from the post-enumeration program and from the 1980 Housing Unit Enumeration Duplication Study suggest, however, that a considerable proportion of the 1980 census count, likely in excess of 1 percent, represented duplicate enumerations of individuals. An additional factor contributing to the improvements in coverage in 1980 is the appropriate counting of a significant number of illegal aliens for the first time ever. The Census Bureau estimates the inclusion of 2.06 million undocumented residents.

Analyses indicate that coverage completeness in 1990 was less than that of the 1980 census. As noted by Passel (1993), however, evidence suggests that improvements in 1990 census operations led to fewer duplications than in 1980, with a resulting *increase* in net undercount rates.

Studies which investigated the completeness of coverage and the accuracy of characteristics in the death registration were also reviewed. While coverage in the death registration data is generally assumed to be practically complete, no national test of its completeness has been conducted since completion of the Death Registration Area in 1933. Coale and Kisker (1990) suggest, however, that under-registration of deaths exists, particularly at older ages and for the African American population.

Evaluations of the quality of characteristic (age, race, and sex) reporting have also been sparse in the literature. Five major studies have analyzed the quality of death certificate characteristics by linking the death certificate to an independent data source. Poe et al (1992) linked death certificates selected from the 1986 Current Mortality Sample (CMS) to responses on the 1986 National Mortality Followback Survey (NMFS), a nationally representative (except Oregon) sample that questioned the death certificate informant within one year following the death of an adult in 1986. Sorlie et al (1992) evaluated the validity of race and sex characteristics by linkage of the Current Population Survey to the National Death Index. Kestenbaum (1990; no date) linked death certificates from Texas and Massachusetts to improved social security/Medicare administrative records for the elderly population. Rosenwaike and Logue (1983) matched death certificates for the population aged 85 and over in the 1968 to 1972 period to the 1900 manuscript of population. And, Hambright (NCHS,

Adjustments to the Data Sources

1968; Hambright, 1969) matched a national sample of death certificates from May to August 1960 with the 1960 census records.

The linked studies, while clearly highlighting inconsistencies between the reporting of characteristics in two independent data sources, fail to determine which data set reports "true" age, if either. Nonetheless, two general conclusions were reached based on these studies. First, there is lower percentage agreement between the sources for old-age African Americans relative to whites. Second, the levels of agreement decrease as age advances. Only the Hambright study compared reporting of age in death registration relative to a census at a point in time. For whites of all ages and nonwhites aged less than 45 years, the age reported on the death certificate was, on average, older than that reported on the census. For nonwhites aged 45 and above, however, age reported on the death certificate was younger than on the census.

A brief discussion of net immigration statistics was also provided. While the quality of immigration tabulations in the US is widely acknowledged to be suspect, the estimation of population size at the older ages is quite robust to variations in estimates of intercensal migration. This robustness results both from the greater magnitude of deaths as a source of decrement in the older age groups relative to change as a result of net migration and from the smaller flow of net migrants at the older ages relative to younger ages.

These evaluations highlighted a number of inherent problems in the data sources, including a large overcount of the centenarian population in the 1970 census, racial misclassification in all three population censuses, and low quality in the immigration statistics. The role of this chapter will be to describe adjustments made to the basic data sources and to provide justifications for the changes. The chapter is divided into five major sections. First, we will consider data quality and requisite adjustments to the 1970 census. This will be followed by a discussion of race misclassification and other problems in the 1980 census. The third section details race misclassification and probable age inaccuracies in the 1990 census. The fourth section describes the basic death registration data from the National Center for Health Statistics. And, finally, we describe adjustments to the net immigration data.

ADJUSTMENTS TO THE 1970 CENSUS

Three possible sets of tabulations of the 1970 census are available: (1) the official published counts from the Census Bureau, (2) unpublished adjusted tabulations received from Census, and (3) unpublished adjusted tabulations prepared by Shrestha. The strengths and limitations of the three sets of statistics will be presented in the following sections.

The Official Tabulations

As noted in Chapter 2, the official tabulations of the 1970 population by basic demographic characteristics are presented in *Series B--US Summary of the 1970 Census* (US Bureau of the Census, 1972a). These official enumerations are known to contain a number of major inaccuracies. The first and most serious problem for our investigation of the enumerated old-age population is the conspicuous overstatement of the number of persons aged 100 years or more. Significant inconsistencies in the estimated count have been identified for both sexes and for all race groupings (Siegel, 1974; Siegel and Passel, 1976; US Bureau of the Census, 1974a). Indirect demographic analysis estimates the correct centenarian count to be in the range of 3,000 to 8,000 whereas 106,000 persons were actually enumerated in the open-ended age category (100 and above).

A second problem, though of smaller magnitude, is the result of misclassification of the population by race in the complete-count tabulations. Too many persons were classified as "other races", rather than as white (US Bureau of the Census, 1974a). For the Series C (US Bureau of the Census, 1972b) sample tabulations, an editing procedure transferred an estimated 21,000 persons aged 65 and above from the "other races" category to white.

Finally, the official 1970 legal resident population count for the United States is 203,235,298, as opposed to 203,211,926 as presented in the Series B statistics. The difference, over 23,000, represents corrections for errors in the population counts of local areas which were discovered after the initial tabulations were published (US Bureau of the Census, 1974). The age distribution of the 23,000 individuals is not available.

Unpublished adjusted tabulations from the Census Bureau

Because of the inherent errors in the official 1970 census enumeration, unpublished adjusted tabulations were obtained from the Census Bureau. The modifications include correction for the three previously mentioned problems as well as for geocoding, which added an additional 67,000 individuals to the final total census count.

The adjusted statistics improve on the published statistics for a number of reasons. First, without modification, the excess number of centenarians is sufficiently large to bias research results at the oldest ages. Furthermore, it appears that the overcount of centenarians was due to a misunderstanding of the census form wherein individuals confused the columns intended for month of birth and year of birth, rather than from a systematic introduction of bias (Siegel, 1974).

To estimate the correct size of the race- and sex-specific centenarian population in the United States in 1970, the US Bureau of the Census employed forward survival techniques. The 1960 population was survived forward using 1959-61 life table rates. Since the overcount did not appear to have been the result of systematic misreporting of age, the Census Bureau was able to employ a reasonable assumption to distribute the excess centenarians. To maintain the enumerated distribution of individuals, the excess centenarians were allocated *pro rata* for each sex-race group over the entire age distribution under age 100 (Siegel, 1974). The assumption is justified by the belief that the errors in the centenarian enumeration are randomly distributed with respect to age and sex within races. Less information is available about the procedures employed by the Census Bureau to rectify the remaining three problems: race misclassification, omitted individuals, and geocoding errors. First, regarding the race misclassification, the Census Bureau transferred 327,000 persons (of which 21,000 were aged 65 and above) from "unspecified races" to white. The effect on the black count was deemed minimal and no adjustment was made. The transfer methodology is described by Siegel (1974, page 6):

> The age-sex distribution assigned to the reclassified population has been "built up" from [Series B, official] census data on the age-sex distribution of the "other races" population in each county for which a race adjustment had been made.

Second, the 23,000 (at all ages) individuals originally excluded from the tabulations were assigned by sex, race, and age "according to the probable basis of the error" (Siegel, 1974, page 6). Finally, an additional 67,000 persons were added to the final modified file, the result of geocoding (Robinson, 1992).

Tabulations produced by Shrestha

While the official tabulations of the 1970 census greatly overstate the number of centenarians in the US population, the procedures employed by the US Bureau of the Census in the calculation of the unpublished adjusted estimates are likely to have *under*estimated the true population aged 100 and over. The procedure employed was to forward project the 1960 population using 1959-61 life table survival rates. This approach can be expected to underestimate the 1970 centenarian population for two reasons. First, further decreases in mortality in the decade following 1959-61 would cause the 1959-61 survival rates to overestimate the number of deaths in the decade. More importantly, because the US official life tables at the oldest ages for 1959-61 are based on the experience of Civil War veterans, "with improvements in medical technology and care for the aged, it is possible that mortality of the extreme aged has decreased and that survival rates have increased" (Siegel and Passel, 1976:561).

To estimate the "correct" size of the race- and sex-specific centenarian population in the United States in 1970, Siegel and Passel (ibid) employed various methodologies, including: (1) comparison with tabulations of Medicare records, (2) survival from prior censuses, and (3) population reconstruction using deaths. The calculated estimates are presented in Table 4.1

Table 4.1
Alternative Estimates of Population Aged 100 & Over, by Sex and Race: April 1, 1970

Estimation Method	All Classes	Whites Males	Whites Females	Blacks & Others Males	Blacks & Others Females
		Number			
Census Count[1]	106,441	46,015	42,965	8,323	9,138
Medicare Records[2]	7,341	1,508	4,209	513	1,111
Forward Survival					
From 1960 with 1959-61 life table rates	3,395	1,109	1,985	121	180
From 1960 with Medicare rates	7,713	1,606	4,263	651	1,193
From 1950 with 1949-51/1959-61 l.t. rates	3,222	1,090	1,795	136	201
Population reconstruction[3]					
Stationary Assumption	8,211	1,387	3,957	958	1,909
Least Squares	7,854	1,441	4,173	661	1,579
Preferred Estimate	**4,800**	**1,250**	**2,650**	**300**	**600**

Table 4.1 (*continued*), in Percent

Estimation Method	All Classes	Whites Males	Whites Females	Blacks & Others Males	Blacks & Others Females
Census Count[1]	100.0	43.2	40.4	7.8	8.6
Medicare Records[2]	100.0	20.5	57.4	7.0	15.1
Forward Survival					
From 1960 with 1959-61 life table rates	100.0	32.7	58.5	3.6	5.3
From 1960 with Medicare rates	100.0	20.8	55.3	8.4	15.5
From 1950 with 1949-51/1959-61 l.t. rates	100.0	33.8	55.7	4.2	6.2
Population reconstruction[3]					
Stationary Assumption	100.0	16.9	48.2	11.7	23.2
Least Squares	100.0	18.3	53.1	8.4	20.1
Preferred Estimate	**100.0**	**26.0**	**55.2**	**5.2**	**12.5**

Source: Siegel, J.S. & J.S. Passel, 1976. New estimates of the number of centenarians in the United States. *Demography*, 71(355):559-566, Table 1.
Notes: (1) As enumerated in 1970 census. (2) Persons whose race or sex were not reported have been distributed *pro rata*; figures include 1,029 persons whose race was not reported and 5 persons whose race and sex were not reported; (3) For Jan. 1, 1970; (4) Fitted equations used 4 data points except for Negro-and-others (2 points).

Rather than to estimate the "correct" size of the centenarian population, our goal was to estimate the number of individuals aged 100 and over that would have been enumerated in the 1970 census in the absence of the misunderstanding of the census questionnaire. We utilize estimates of the Medicare population to accomplish this task. Our choice was based on research by Coale and Kisker (1990), who found the Medicare population to be of the same general magnitude and subject to the same "normal" biases (i.e., not associated with the 1970 Census questionnaire format) as found in Census records. Estimates of the Medicare centenarian population as of April 1, 1970 were provided by Siegel and Passel (1976) by race and sex. We utilize their estimates of the white centenarian population (see Table 4.2), without adjustment. Since estimates of the black centenarian population are included in a "black and other races" category in the Siegel and Passel publication, a minor adjustment was required. We estimated the proportion black of all nonwhites in the centenarian population by sex, based on that proportion in the 1970 census. Note that, although the centenarian population in 1970 is greatly overstated, the proportion black of all nonwhites is very similar to the same proportion as enumerated for the 1980 centenarian population. Therefore, the proportion was then applied to Siegel and Passel's estimate of the number of "black and other races" Medicare enrollees by sex. Using this methodology, we calculated 453 black males and 1003 black female centenarians. Although the number of both whites and blacks aged 100 and over in the Medicare data (and hence in our estimates) is likely overstated, we believe that these numbers approximate the number of centenarians that would have been enumerated in the absence of misunderstanding of the census form. In all likelihood, the remaining inflation in the centenarian population is due to age misreporting.

Table 4.2

Various Estimates of US Population in the 1970 Census, by Race, Sex, and Age

		Adjusted Tabulations (Census)	Published Tabulations (Census)	Adjusted Tabulations (Shrestha)
ALL AGES	Total	203,302,031	203,211,926	203,211,926
	Wh M	86,934,629	86,720,987	86,720,987
	Wh F	91,220,337	91,027,988	91,027,988
	Bl M	10,752,676	10,748,316	10,748,316
	Bl F	11,836,047	11,831,973	11,831,973
	Ot M	1,271,857	1,442,889	1,442,889
	Ot F	1,286,485	1,439,773	1,439,773
AGES 60 & OVER	Total	28,605,551	28,682,286	----NC----
	Wh M	11,273,504	11,292,918	11,254,186
	Wh F	14,826,286	14,842,134	14,809,682
	Bl M	1,003,648	1,009,995	1,003,745
	Bl F	1,275,620	1,282,536	1,276,073
	Ot M	123,687	139,767	----NC----
	Ot F	102,806	114,936	----NC----

To maintain the enumerated distribution of individuals, we allocated the excess centenarians by race and sex *pro rata*, justified by our belief that the inaccuracies found in the centenarian population were randomly distributed, with respect to age and sex within races. The Shrestha tabulations do not adjust for the three additional problems associated with the 1970 census: racial misclassification, omitted individuals, and geocoding errors.

Data Source Utilized in this Book

Because of the inherent errors in the official census enumeration, use of unpublished adjusted tabulations of the 1970 census are warranted in this book. Although the Shrestha estimates of the centenarian population are plausibly closest to that which would have been enumerated in the absence of misunderstanding of the 1970 census questionnaire, they fail to correct for other identified problems in the official statistics at other ages, including racial misclassification, errors in the population counts of local areas, and geocoding errors. For this reason, unpublished adjusted estimates obtained from the US Bureau of the Census are utilized in this book. As discussed earlier, however, these estimates likely underestimate the number of centenarians in the 1970 census. A sensitivity analysis, which compares the results of intercensal cohort analysis to the differing 1970 census estimates, was conducted. The principal conclusion was that the intercensal results of observed/expected population are highly insensitive to the choice of adjusted 1970 census estimates. Because the population aged 100 and over in 1980 is estimated by the forward survival of the population aged *90 and over* in 1970, relatively small differences in the centenarian estimates are diluted by the absolute size of the population aged 90 and above in 1970.

ADJUSTMENTS TO THE 1980 CENSUS[1]

Race Misclassification: transferring an overcount in the "other, not specified" race category to specified races

Originally published census tabulations for 1980 were presented in *Series B--US Summary of the 1980 Census* (US Bureau of the Census, 1983a). Data on race were provided by responses to Question 4 on the census questionnaire. Fourteen categories of race were designated as precoded response categories: (1) White, (2) Black/Negro, (3) American Indian, (4) Eskimo, (5) Aleut, (6) Japanese, (7) Chinese, (8) Filipino, (9) Korean, (10) Vietnamese, (11) Asian Indian, (12) Hawaiian, (13) Guamanian, and, (14) Samoan. From these groupings, responses could be unambiguously condensed into the four major race groups specified by the Office of Management and Budget (White; Black; American Indian/Alaskan Native; and Asian or Pacific Islander) (US Bureau of the Census, 1983b).

In the 1980 census, however, a large number (about 6.76 million) of individuals enumerated chose to write-in a response to the race question as opposed to selecting one of the specified all-inclusive race categories. Referring to Table 4.3, a large proportion (86%) of these individuals were of Hispanic origin.

Table 4.3

Racial Identification in the 1980 Census

226,545,805 persons were enumerated, of which:

219,787,486 (97%) chose one of the 14 specified response categories.	6,758,319 (3%) were enumerated in the "other, not specified" category. These persons replied with write-in responses.	
	Hispanic-Origin: 5,841,810 (86%) were allocated to only the white & black categories.	Not of Hispanic-Origin: 916,509 (14%) were distributed to white, black, and "other" (American Indian/Asian/ Pacific Islander)

Source: US Bureau of the Census, 1983. Census of Population: 1980. *County population by age, sex, race, and Spanish origin (preliminary OMB-consistent modified race)*. Wash., DC: Technical Documentation: Attach. 4: pp. 1-13.

Data are presented in its unmodified form in the 1980 census publications, summary tape files, and public use samples. (Note, however, that more detailed and careful editing and coding of responses in the sample processing may have transferred individuals from the "other, not specified" category to specified races). All 6.76 million individuals with write-in responses are included in the residual "other races" (other than the 14 specified races) category. Originally

Adjustments to the Data Sources

published census tabulations for 1980, hence, were not directly comparable with other data sources since only the census enumeration contained a residual racial category. Therefore, to allow comparison with other systems, the Census Bureau was compelled to modify the 1980 enumerations to conform to historical categories of the racial groupings. The modification, done on the macro-level, involved the reassignment of race for persons in the "other, not specified" category based on detailed cross-tabulations of race and Hispanic origin from the sample and complete-count census data (Robinson, Word, and Spencer, 1991). As shown in Table 4.4, the redistribution of individuals from the "other races, not specified" category to one of the specified categories added 6.351 million persons, or 3.3%, to the white category and 177,000, or 0.7%, to the black population. The other (specified) races category, which consists of American Indians, Alaska Natives, Asians, and Pacific Islanders, will not be explored indepth in this study. The category decreased by 6.5 million (55.9%). As part of the modifications, the population aged 60 and over was also affected, but to a lesser extent. About 141,000 persons were added to the white male category. About 174,000 individuals were added to the white female group. To the black male and female categories were added 4,000 and 6,000, respectively.

The specifics of the modification follow. For the 219.8 million individuals who chose one of the 14 specified categories, no adjustment was made. Two categories of individuals, totalling 6.7 million, with write-in responses were identified: persons of Hispanic-origin (5.8 million) and persons not of Hispanic-origin (0.9 million). Separate adjustment procedures for the two groups were developed.

Those of Hispanic-origin were distributed only to the white or black categories (and not to American Indian or Asian/Pacific Islander categories). All persons of Mexican origin were reassigned as white. Persons of Puerto Rican, Cuban, and other Spanish origin were assigned to both white and black modified race groups on the basis of the distribution of the same Hispanic origin individuals who originally specified either a white or black race on the Census returns. The calculations were carried out within age-sex-county cells.

Those not of Hispanic-origin were reassigned to all three modified race groups (white, black, other (Asian, Pacific Islander, American Indian)) on the basis of state-specific proportions which are applied to all age-sex-county cells within the state. The proportions are based on sample data from the 1980 census.[2]

Table 4.4

Published & Modified Estimates of US Population in 1980 Census, by Race, Sex, and Age

		Modified Counts	Published Tabulations	Difference
ALL AGES	Total	226,545,805	226,545,805	0
	Wh M	94,930,324	91,685,333	3,244,991
	Wh F	99,793,983	96,686,289	3,107,694
	Bl M	12,606,609	12,519,189	87,420
	Bl F	14,065,511	13,975,836	89,675
	Ot M	2,516,228	5,848,639	-3,332,411
	Ot F	2,633,150	5,830,519	-3,197,369
AGES 60 & OVER	Total	35,637,048	35,637,048	0
	Wh M	13,535,783	13,395,175	140,608
	Wh F	18,702,707	18,528,729	173,978
	Bl M	1,235,743	1,231,764	3,979
	Bl F	1,732,063	1,725,930	6,133
	Ot M	203,281	347,868	-144,587
	Ot F	227,471	407,582	-180,111

Sources: (1) US Bureau of the Census, 1983. Census of Population: 1980. *Characteristics of the Population*. Vol. 1. PC80-1-B1. Table 41; (2) US Bureau of the Census, 1983a. Census of Population: 1980. *General Population Characteristics*. Final Report PC80-1-B1. United States Summary. Washington, D.C.: US Government Printing Office; (3) US Bureau of the Census, 1984b. Census of Population: 1980. Race Detail File. 100% Count. Table IV: modified counts (OMB-consistent) by age, race, and sex. Unpublished tabulations. Computer run dated 9/7/84.

The decision was made to use the race-modified statistics for this research. For the white population, the decision was clear-cut because of the sheer magnitude of the transfers. If we were to use the unmodified numbers, we would omit 6.351 million individuals from the white tabulations, of which 315,000 were aged 60 and above. For the black population, however, the judgment to use race-modified statistics was made with much hesitancy. Their use was favored by the large number of blacks erroneously included in the "unspecified other races" category in the unmodified statistics. For the total black population, this number equalled 177,000, of which 10,000 were aged 60 and above. On the other hand, a change in Census Bureau procedures in allocating race for persons of Puerto Rican and Cuban ethnicity was noted. Although the race modification procedures were intended to increase the comparability of the 1980 census enumerations to earlier censuses and to other data collection systems, classification of these individuals in the modified 1980 statistics became less consistent with the other sources. In the earlier censuses *and in the vital registration system*, for Puerto Ricans and Cubans without a specified racial classification, allocation was made to the white category. In the 1980 modification procedures, however, these individuals were allocated to white and black according to the racial distribution of that ethnicity in the enumerated population. For example, we estimate that about 24,850 (or about 5.15%) of the 483,015 Puerto Rican-born individuals with write-in responses had been transferred to the black category. In the 1970 census and in the vital registration system, these persons would have been identified as "white."

Another Race-Related Problem in the 1980 Census

Aside from the issue of racial modification due to write-in responses, another race-related issue exists in the 1980 census. "Asian Indian" was added as a separate response category to the race question. This category is included in the "Asian and Pacific Islander" grouping or the "other races" category in 1980 census tabulations. In past censuses and in vital statistics through 1978, persons of Asian Indian descent were classified as "white." This group numbered 362,000 in 1980, but was much smaller, probably less than 100,000, in 1970 (US Bureau of the Census, 1988). In our procedures, no adjustment was made for the reclassification of Asian Indians for two reasons. First, we believe that only relatively small numbers of individuals were affected at the oldest ages. Second, an age and sex distribution of the 1980 Asian Indian population is not available.

Overcount of Centenarians in the 1980 Census

As noted in Chapter 2, the centenarian population in 1980 is believed to be overcounted due to Census Bureau procedures used to allocate age. While 24,000 individuals self-reported an age of 100 or over, an additional 8,000 reached this position by allocation (US Bureau of the Census, 1983b). In our procedures, no adjustment is made for the centenarian overcount.

ADJUSTMENTS TO THE 1990 CENSUS

As was the case with the earlier censuses, the published statistics from the 1990 census contain a number of problems that make comparability to earlier censuses and to other sources of data (vital registration, immigration, etc.) difficult. Three problems are apparent: racial misclassification, inconsistencies in the reporting of age, and a change in allocation procedures for the 1990 census in assigning age to persons with missing data on the characteristic.

A modified 1990 census file, referred to as the MARS (Modified Age and Race Statistics) was produced at the Census Bureau to adjust for the first two problems. As in 1980, the race statistics were modified "to be consistent with the classification used in data systems other than the census" (Word and Spencer, 1991). The age data were adjusted to correspond with the April 1, 1990 census date. A comparison of the published and modified population counts by selected population characteristics is presented in Table 4.5.

Table 4.5

Published & Modified Estimates of US Population in 1990 Census, by Race, Sex, and Age

		Modified Counts	Published Tabulations	Difference
ALL AGES	Total	248,709,873	248,709,873	0
	Wh M	102,142,817	97,475,880	4,666,937
	Wh F	106,561,348	102,210,190	4,351,158
	Bl M	14,420,331	14,170,151	250,180
	Bl F	16,062,950	15,815,909	247,041
	Ot M	4,676,200	9,593,337	-4,917,137
	Ot F	4,846,227	9,444,356	-4,598,129
AGES 60 & OVER	Total	41,704,104	41,857,998	-153,894
	Wh M	15,693,394	15,549,693	143,701
	Wh F	21,707,770	21,513,403	194,367
	Bl M	1,375,083	1,379,677	-4,594
	Bl F	2,088,898	2,090,493	-1,595
	Ot M	370,943	582,850	-211,907
	Ot F	468,016	741,882	-273,866

Source: Derived from Word, David L. and Gregory Spencer, 1991. Age, sex, race, and Hispanic origin information from the 1990 census: a comparison of census results with results where age and race have been modified. File 1990 CPH-L-74. Draft dated August, 1991.

Details of the Race Modification

Fifteen specific racial categories were listed on the census form. A significant number of individuals, however, chose to write-in a response to the race question instead of choosing one of the specified categories. The problem affected the enumeration of 9.8 million persons. (A similar problem in the 1980 census enumeration affected 6.8 million individuals). Over 95% percent of the total "other race" persons are individuals of Hispanic origin who reported their race on the census form as "Mexican", "Puerto Rican", etc. (Hollmann and Spencer, 1992a). Since such "non-specified other race" persons are not found in data sources other than the census, a modification procedure was developed to transfer them to the specified categories.

Unlike in 1980, when a macro-level reassignment of race based on detailed cross-tabulations of race and Hispanic origin from the sample and complete-count census data were employed, the 1990 modification procedure was conducted at the micro-level. Hot-deck imputation procedures are utilized to assign a specific race to persons who reported themselves in the "other, not specified" racial category. The method was executed on the individual records of the 100% edited detail file from the 1990 census (Robinson, Word, and Spencer, 1991). After evaluating many alternatives (some of which are described in Robinson, Word, and Spencer, 1991), the following features were chosen for the reassignment methodology:

1. The Hispanic origin response of each "other race" person was taken into account when assigning a specified race. This procedure is similar to that used in creating the modified-race file in 1980. It is appropriate because 97.5 percent of those without a specified race in 1990 were of Hispanic origin. Their origin response was used, whether or not it had been allocated, in order to preserve the race distribution within each type of origin. The specific Hispanic origin responses were "not Spanish/Hispanic, Mexican, Puerto Rican, Cuban, and other Spanish/Hispanic".

2. Virtually all persons who reported both a specified race and an origin were included in the "donor pool" from which each of the 9.8 million "other races" were assigned a race. The sole exception was the exclusion of several American

Indian codes from the donor pool " . . . because these codes represent general responses rather than true tribal answers."

3. The assignment of a specified race was made on an individual basis. That is, no attempt was made to minimize racial heterogeneity within households. Any such attempt would have made it difficult to assign race in a manner which approximated the specified-race distribution reported by persons with the same Hispanic origin response. Furthermore, it is not at all clear that racial heterogeneity should be minimized within these households.

4. Special procedures were adopted for the "hot deck" matrices to minimize distortions produced by unusually low ratios of donors to donees in these matrices. Typically, real data from donors are stored in hot decks far more frequently than the data needed by persons without the characteristic (the donees). In this file, conversely, there were a number of occasions where those needing a specified race outnumbered those of the same origin with a specified race.

This problem was ameliorated by expanding the allocation matrices so that each cell held 64 values (rather than the typical 8 used in most census matrices). The initial race data in these 64 cells were then obtained by loading real data ("warming" the hot deck) before doing the race assignments. Finally, the actual allocation was performed by random assignment from the 64 values (none was used more than once until all had been used at least once).

The procedures differ from those utilized in the 1980 race reassignment in two important aspects. First, the 1990 reassignment was done on a micro-level whereas the 1980 transfer was performed on the macro-level. Second, in the 1990 procedures, those of Mexican origin could be transferred to the white, black, or other races categories, based on the racial distribution of the Mexican origin population. In contrast, Mexicans were assigned only to the white category in both 1970 and 1980.

Details of the Census Bureau's Age Modification (Hollmann and Spencer, 1992a; Word and Spencer, 1991)

Although "the data appear reasonable for virtually every age and 93% of the respondents appeared to have perfect data, i.e. their age and year of birth responses were consistent" (Hollmann and Spencer, 1992a), a decision was made at the Census Bureau to modify the age characteristics of the enumerated population. The judgment was based on two findings in detailed review of the 1990 information. First, some respondents provided their age as of the date of completion of the questionnaire, not their age as of April 1, 1990. Word (1993) has speculated that this problem particularly affects those individuals with two characteristics. First, they were counted after April 1 in a follow-up interview by Census enumerators due to non-response to the mail questionnaire. Second, they had a birthday between the April 1 census date and the personal interview. In addition to this problem, there may have been a tendency for respondents to round up their age if they were close to having a birthday. Approximately 10% of persons in most age groups are estimated to be one year younger. For most single years of age, the misstatements are largely offsetting. The problem is most pronounced at age 0 because persons lost to age 1 may not have been fully offset by the inclusion of babies born after April 1, 1990, and because there may have been more rounding up to age 1 to avoid reporting age as 0 years.

The inconsistencies in the reporting in age between the earlier censuses (1970 and 1980) and that of 1990 may be the result of a change in the "age" question on the 1990 census questionnaire. Respondents in both 1970 and 1980 were requested to: (1) print age at last birthday and to (2) both print and provide responses for month and year of birth in FOSDIC-readable form. In 1990, in contrast, respondents were asked to provide only age and year of birth (in both print and FOSDIC-readable form). Month or quarter of birth was not requested. Note that the specific age question in all three census years asked only for "age at last birthday," without reference to the census date of April 1.

Although about 95% of the population in 1990 provided acceptable birth year responses, the following procedures were utilized to adjust the data (taken directly from Hollmann and Spencer, 1992a and Word and Spencer, 1991:II):

The age data for individuals in households were modified by adjusting the reported birth year data by race and sex for each of the 1990 Census' 449 district offices to correspond with the national level quarterly distribution of births available from the National Center for Health Statistics. The data for persons in groups quarters were adjusted on a state basis to minimize the number of matrix cells with very small numbers. The central assumption in this procedure is that there is not reason for the residents of any sub-national area to have a different quarter of birth distribution from that found at the national level. It was also assumed that there are no significant birth place-sex-race-origin differences in annual birth distributions by quarter, that all those born before 1920 have the same quarter of birth distribution, and that mortality is not selective by quarter of birth. *Approximately 100 million persons* (emphasis added) have an age in this modified file which is one year different from that they had in the 1990 census. The modification procedure was done separately for each birth year, by sex, for the white, black, Asian or Pacific Islander, and American Indian, Eskimo, or Aleut populations. For every birth year the program was provided with the number of cases out of 10,000 where the birth year plus the person's age should equal 1989. These overall control values were calculated from the available monthly birth statistics for the 1920 to 1989 period. Earlier birth years were each assumed to have the same seasonal pattern as was exhibited by the unweighted average of the 1920-24 birth cohorts. Each sex-race-origin cell was next randomly assigned a value of 0, 0.25, 0.5, or 0.75. Then, each time that birth year cell was encountered, a test was made to see if that birth year plus the person's age should equal 1989 or 1990. The choice of an age was dependent on whether its acceptance moved the cell's actual population distribution toward the control value distribution.

Justification for Use of Modified 1990 Census Data

The relevant issue for this book was whether to use the unmodified statistics from published sources or to use the MARS (modified age and race statistics) file available from the Census Bureau. Again, because of the magnitude of persons (9.8 million in the total population) who did not choose one of the specified races, use of the unmodified statistics would seriously bias estimates of the white population. Furthermore, in 1990, the size of the transfer to the black population approximated one-half million individuals, as opposed to in 1980 when smaller numbers were transferred to the black count. For the 1990 population aged 60 and above, the race and age modifications added 338,000 individuals to the white category, but reduced both the black (by 6,200) and the other races (by 486,000) classifications. In addition, use of the race modified file is consistent with use of the 1980 modified statistics in this book. While use of the race modifications is judged valuable for this book, justification for utilization of the age modifications is lacking.

Although the age problem was gauged to be serious only at age 0, "approximately 100 million persons have an age in this modified file which is one year different from that they had in the 1990 census" (Hollmann and Spencer, 1992a). In our judgment, such a massive age modification is unjustified. First, although the census age question changed in 1990, there was no evidence to support the notion that respondents in 1990 behaved differently in their approach to the enumeration date of April 1st relative to earlier census years. Second, although the Census Bureau estimates that about ten percent of persons in most age groups are actually one year younger, a monumental 100 million persons (or 40.2 percent of the total enumerated population) have a different age in the modified file relative to enumerated age. And, finally, in the modification procedure, it was assumed that "there are no significant birth place-sex-race-origin differences in annual birth distributions by quarter, that all those born before 1920 have the same quarter of birth distribution, and that mortality is not selective by quarter of birth." No discussion of the effects of the likely violation of the assumptions was presented. Unfortunately, however, a separate race-modified file is not available from the Census Bureau. Instead only a file which adjusts for both race and age exists. Despite the encumbrances of the age modification, we believe that the MARS file provides a more accurate description of the 1990 population. Use of unmodified statistics would seriously bias the age-specific count and the racial distribution of the population, particularly for whites. A sensitivity analysis, which compares the results of intercensal cohort analysis to the modified and unmodified estimates in 1980 and 1990, was conducted. The principal conclusion is that the pattern of the results is highly insensitive to the choice between modified or unmodified estimates, for both the African

American and the white populations. The magnitude of the results, however, is slightly dependent on the decision.

THE VITAL REGISTRATION SYSTEM

National-level annual death statistics from the National Center for Health Statistics (NCHS) have been utilized for this research project. The data for 1970 through 1988 are extracted from NCHS data tapes where data are available by single years of age to an open-ended category at age 125 (NCHS, 1970-1988). The data for 1989 and the first three months of 1990 are from the Advance Reports on Mortality (NCHS, 1989; NCHS, 1990; NCHS, 1992) with adjustments as described below.

Adjustments have been made for neither under-registration of deaths nor for misreporting of characteristics on the death certificates. Two problems were noted that affected the utilization of our intended intercensal methodology. First, the intercensal period covers the interval from April 1st to March 31st, whereas the published death registration data refer to calendar years. Therefore, annual deaths in the intercensal period were adjusted for the timing of the census.

Second, both the death registration and the US censuses' data are reported by age at last birthday rather than by year of birth. Because the census is on April 1, the latter is preferred because it identifies the birth cohort for use in cohort analysis.

To adjust for these two problems, i.e. of adjusting deaths to the same intercensal period as dictated by census dates and of relating deaths and census counts to the appropriate birth cohort, the following procedure, as illustrated by Table 4.6 was used. We used available data to estimate separation factors that reflect the distribution of deaths in a census calendar year at age i and $i+1$ to appropriate birth cohorts.

These categories identify those deaths reported in the one year interval between census date April 1, 1970 and March 31, 1971, to those aged 60 (last birthday) at the time of the census. Note, however, that those deaths occurred in both 1970 and 1971, and that they occurred to persons aged 60 and 61 (last birthday).

Table 4.6

Deaths in Parallelogram between April 1, 1970 and April 1, 1971

Category	Age (Last Birthday)	Calendar Year	Proportion
1	60	1970	15/32
2	60	1971	1/32
3	61	1970	9/32
4	61	1971	7/32

Persons were differentiated into four classifications based on these characteristics, and the proportion in each category was calculated. In making these assignments, we have assumed that the three dimensional surface of the number of deaths in age and time is level over the interval. Because NCHS data tapes provide a variable for month of death, we were able to refine the above procedure. We were able to calculate the number of deaths by single years of age, race, and sex for two time periods: (1) April 1 up to January 1, and (2) January 1 up to April 1. In our example, deaths that occurred in 1970 (April 1 up to January 1) were at two ages (last birthday): 60 and 61. The number of deaths at age 60 is calculated as: the number of deaths from April 1 up to January 1 multiplied by the proportion 15/24. Similarly, to estimate the number of deaths at age 61, we multiply the number of deaths from April 1 up to January 1 by 9/24. A similar procedure is used to allocate the deaths from January 1 up to April 1 to ages 60 and 61. The relevant separation factors are 1/8 and 7/8 respectively. Application of the intercensal cohort method required the use of these complex proportions of deaths for correct projection of the population aged i and above forward.

Estimates of Mortality in 1989 and 1990

Since the NCHS data tapes for 1989 and 1990 had yet to be released, a procedure to estimate the death distribution in these years was developed. Final mortality statistics for 1989 by race and sex were released in published form in NCHS (1992). The grouped age data was distributed to single years of age based on the 1988 death distribution within the grouped age category. Estimates of the death distribution in 1990 are based on monthly advance reports of mortality from NCHS (1990). Note that death statistics are only required for January, February, and March 1990 since the intercensal period extends only up to April 1, 1990. The preliminary numbers were distributed to single years of age again using the 1988 distribution within the grouped age category.

NET IMMIGRATION STATISTICS

The intercensal cohort methodology utilized in this book requires use of an accurate net immigration series or immigration assumption to estimate the population at a subsequent time. Yet, as noted in Chapter 3, the lack of accurate and timely information on net immigration matters is widely acknowledged (Panel on Immigration Statistics, 1985). The US Bureau of the Census, while not mandated to collect immigration statistics, compiles and corrects a wide variety of information on the flow and stock of migrants due to its need for immigration data for current population estimation and projection. We will rely heavily on these unpublished tabulations, which are the only known series of net immigration statistics available for the US population by net immigration component, age, race, and sex.

While the quality of immigration statistics in the United States is suspect due to the lack of sufficient collection mechanisms, the estimation of population size at the older ages is quite robust to variations in the estimates of intercensal migration. This is the result of the greater magnitude of deaths as a source of decrement in the older age groups relative to changes as a result of the entrance/exit of immigrants. Furthermore, a smaller quantity of immigrants is observed at older ages relative to younger ages, partly due to the negligible number of immigrants in certain component immigrant categories (e.g., net movement of students, net migration of Armed Forces overseas, etc.).

Table 4.7 presents estimates of components of change (deaths and net immigration) for the elderly population (by race and sex) for the 1970-1980 intercensal period.

Table 4.7
Components of Change in the Estimated Resident Population,
by Race, Sex, and Age (in 1980): Decade Ending April 1, 1980

Component of Change	All Ages	60-64	65-69	70-74	75-79	80-84	85+
White Males							
Deaths (-)	9,329,672	717,963	963,720	1,153,609	1,198,961	1,178,210	2,138,492
Net Immigration (NI)	1,239,447	9,185	2,990	-8,132	-5,953	-6,998	-11,647
Legal Immigr. (+)	1,079,039	17,635	16,073	11,449	7,304	3,361	2,453
Legal Emigr. (-)	522,587	17,650	16,598	21,273	14,385	10,974	14,558
Other Immigr. (+)	682,995	9,200	3,515	1,692	1,128	615	458
Ratio: Deaths to NI	8	78	322	142	201	168	184
White Females							
Deaths (-)	7,607,588	389,903	529,090	688,881	858,013	1,088,416	2,978,996
Net Immigration	216,342	6,397	3,085	-12,811	-19,831	-20,048	-29,910
Legal Immigr. (+)	1,139,141	25,584	23,216	16,608	10,867	5,717	3,845
Legal Emigr. (-)	699,991	26,073	24,805	32,154	21,563	26,900	34,688
Other Immigr. (+)	222,808	6,886	4,674	2,735	1,865	1,135	933
Ratio: Deaths to NI	35	61	172	54	43	54	100

Adjustments to the Data Sources 99

Table 4.7 (*continued*)
Components of Change in the Estimated Resident Population,
by Race, Sex, and Age (in 1980): Decade Ending April 1, 1980

Component of Change	All Ages	60-64	65-69	70-74	75-79	80-84	85+
Black Males							
Deaths (-)	1,263,025	109,630	130,254	137,784	126,259	105,257	150,526
Net Immigration (NI)	186,203	2,831	1,851	832	450	97	64
Legal Immigr. (+)	201,937	3,626	2,637	1,482	798	302	208
Legal Emigr. (-)	55,057	1,281	915	684	343	196	143
Other Immigr. (+)	39,323	486	129	34	-5	-9	-1
Ratio: Deaths to NI	7	39	70	166	281	1,085	2,352
Black Females							
Deaths (-)	974,358	73,247	92,357	105,943	103,293	97,927	196,408
Net Immigration	164,260	3,773	2,965	1,436	679	214	133
Legal Immigr. (+)	218,063	6,071	4,650	2,762	1,576	721	470
Legal Emigr. (-)	72,001	2,509	1,818	1,359	905	512	350
Other Immigr. (+)	18,198	211	133	33	8	5	13
Ratio: Deaths to NI	6	19	31	74	152	458	1,477

Table 4.7 (*continued*)

Source: Unpublished tabulations from the US Bureau of the Census.

Notes: (1) Net immigration totals exclude estimates of net illegal aliens; (2) "Other Immigration" includes net movement of refugees and parolees, civilian citizens, Puerto Ricans, resident foreign students, and the Armed Forces stationed overseas; (3) Ratio, which is used to denote the relative importance of deaths as a component of change, is calculated by dividing deaths by the absolute value of net immigration; (4) - denotes a negative value.

Adjustments to the Data Sources 101

The net immigration data provided by the US Bureau of the Census were categorized in the form of "Components of Change" for each of the two decades. The various categories (listed below) of immigration data, tabulated by race, sex, and five-year age group, allowed construction of a net immigration series that reflects changes in the US resident population due to in- and out-flows of migrants.

For this book, age-, race-, and sex-specific net immigration was calculated on a cohort basis by use of the following equation (4.1):

> Net Immigration = Legal Alien Immigration + Refugees and Parolees + Net Civilian Citizens Immigration + Net Puerto Rican Immigration + Net Foreign Students Immigration + Net Movement of US Armed Forces Overseas - Legal Emigration

Estimates of the flow of undocumented residents are not included in the constructed immigration series, but will be considered in the interpretation of results. Their exclusion was precipitated by two factors. First, in the old-age categories, even the most exaggerated estimates of the number of illegal aliens are small relative to the number of deaths as a source of change in the composition of the cohorts. Second, estimates of the magnitude and of the characteristic distribution of the illegal population vary widely due to insufficient data collection instruments in the United States. Because of the uncertainty, the Census Bureau (1988) presented estimates of the 1980 census population under varying assumptions regarding the undocumented population, with estimates ranging from 0 (legally resident population only) to 5 million for the total population. For the population aged 60 and above in 1980, the Census Bureau estimates range from 0 to 93 thousand (all races and sexes). Hill (1985) summarized the findings of major studies (listed in Chapter 3) which evaluated the size of the illegal population, or components thereof, since the early 1970s. Reiterating from Chapter 3, his review concludes that: (1) variations from method to method are large, (2) the estimates do not show a clear trend over time, (3) for those studies that produced estimates of upper and lower population limits, the range between the limits is typically large, (4) the procedures used all invoke assumptions that often cannot be adequately justified and to which the estimates obtained are sensitive, and (5) the commonly quoted range of 3-6 million illegals may be too high.

Adjustments to the Immigration Data

Given the lack of sufficient detail in the raw data provided by the US Census Bureau, a number of adjustments were required. Details of the following modifications follow: dividing of the open-ended terminal age group into five-year groups, converting the data from its five-year age grouping (to age 100) into single years of age by the use of osculatory interpolation, and creation of an estimate for Puerto Rican immigration during the 1980 to 1990 intercensal period.

Treatment of the Terminal Age Group

The first modification involved dividing the open-ended terminal group into five-year age groups. The data had been provided with 75 and over (age at the beginning of the decade) as the open-ended interval, whereas use of intercensal cohort methodology (in Chapter 5) would be enhanced by an open-ended interval beginning at age 100. To distribute to the five-year age groupings, we assumed that the age-, race- and sex- specific net immigration rate for ages 75+, calculated by dividing net immigration by the mid-decade population, remained constant in the open-ended interval beginning at age 75. This admittedly crude estimate is adequate because of the small numbers of net immigrants in this age group, particularly for the black populations, and because of the relative significance of mortality as a component of change. For example, the net immigration data listed an inflow of 64 black males for the cohort aged 75 and above in 1970 during the 1970 to 1980 decade. For comparison, over 141,000 deaths were recorded for the same cohort. For white males, an outflow of 11,647 migrants was recorded, relative to almost 2,115,000 decrements due to mortality.

Converting the five-year data into single-years of age

The second major adjustment involved converting the data from its five-year age grouping (to age 100) into single years of age by the use of osculatory interpolation, following procedures as described in Shryock and Siegel (1976). Interpolation refers to the inference of unknown values in a particular series of numbers at points intermediate between given values using either graphical or mathematical techniques (Pressat, 1988; Shryock and Siegel, 1976). One such mathematical procedure is to assume that the series of numbers follows an equation (4.2) of the general form,

$$y = A + Bx + Cx^2 + Dx^3 \ldots,$$

a polynomial of the *nth* degree which can be passed through *n+1* given points. As shown, the equation represents a cubic, which can be passed through four known points. With use of single polynomial interpolation formulas, however, breaks in the values of first-order differences may occur at points where two interpolation curves meet. Osculatory interpolation, a procedure which merges overlapping polynomials into a single equation, was consequently developed to allow a smooth nexus where curves meet. An assortment of osculatory interpolation equations exist, varying in the number of terms used, the differences to be minimized, the degree of smoothing or graduation of the given values, and data requirements. To sub-divide our data from five-year age groups to single years of age, we rely upon the Sprague formula (see Shyrock and Siegel, 1976), which is a six-term fifth-difference formula which maintains the given aggregate values. Calculation is eased by the use of Sprague "multipliers", or interpolation coefficients which are based on the Sprague formula.

Creation of Estimates of Puerto Rican Immigration in 1980-90

Because the Census Bureau had not completed its estimates of net Puerto Rican immigration in the 1980 to 1990 intercensal period by the completion of this book, creation of an acceptable proxy was required. I used sex-, race-, and age-specific absolute estimates from the 1970-1980 decade. This admittedly unrefined method is expected to have inconsequential effects in the intercensal computations because of small numbers. For the population aged 60 and above in 1970, an out-migration of only 5,074 whites and 319 blacks was estimated.

As a final note to this chapter, it should be noted that the 1980 to 1990 net immigration estimates received from the Census Bureau and utilized in this book are preliminary.

V

Simulated Effects of Coverage and Age Reporting Errors

This analysis uses intercensal cohort analysis to examine inconsistencies in old-age census and death registration statistics in the United States. The logic of the method is based on the idea that the expected size of an open-ended age cohort in the second census can be estimated from its size at the first census and the intercental deaths occurring to that cohort, after adjustment for migration (Condran, Himes, and Preston, 1991). Because this evaluation is concentrated at the older ages, migration plays only a secondary role relative to decrements from mortality. The methodology is a useful diagnostic tool to identify inconsistencies and possible errors in the data sources. It is not highly precise, however, because different forms of error can produce the same pattern of ratios. Nonetheless, it can help discriminate among competing alternatives.

This chapter will present results of simulations that were carried out in order to evaluate the potential sources of inconsistencies. Simulations of various combinations of coverage completeness and age misreporting patterns in both the census enumerations and the death registration system allows analysis of the effect of the errors on intercensal ratios of observed population at the time of a second census (say, in 1990) to the expected population based on the first (1980) census less intercensal deaths. The principal output of the simulations is the ratio of actual population to expected population at age x at the time of the second census.

In the first section of this chapter, the intercensal cohort methodology will be presented. This will be followed by a discussion of how patterns of age overstatement will affect the age-patterns of the intercensal ratios, based on work by Condran, Himes, and Preston *(ibid)*. The third section will describe procedures used to derive estimates of the "true" 1980 and 1990 population and intercensal death distributions in the United States. The methodology estimates what the "true" distributions would be in the absence of content and age misreporting errors. The fourth section considers the effect of simulated coverage errors in the data sources on the intercensal ratios. Finally, the effects of three types of age reporting on the ratios are considered: accurate reporting, age overstatement, and age understatement.

AN INTERCENSAL METHODOLOGY TO EVALUATE QUALITY OF OLD-AGE DATA

As discussed in the introduction to this chapter, the expected size of an open-ended age cohort in the second census can be estimated from its size at the first census and the intercensal deaths occurring to that cohort, after adjustment for migration (Condran, Himes, and Preston, 1991). Census, death registration, and net immigration data, classified by single years of age, by sex, and by two races (white, black), were utilized to calculate the following refined equation for the expected population at the time of the second census:

$$\hat{N}_x(2) = N_{x-10}(1) - D_{x-10}(1) + M_{x-10}(1) \quad (5.1)$$

where,

$\hat{N}_x(2) =$ the predicted population aged x and above at the second census, taken 10 years after the first.

$N_{x-10}(1) =$ the enumerated population aged x-10 and above at time 1, the first census.

$D_{x-10}(1) =$ the intercensal deaths which had occurred to the cohort aged x-10 and above (at the first census).

$N_{x-10}(1) =$ intercensal net legal immigration into the cohort aged x-10 and above (at the first census).

The expected population *at* a given age (as opposed to at age x and above) can be calculated in an analogous manner. In either circumstance, the ratio of the observed population, enumerated in the subsequent census, to the expected population, can then be calculated (after simplifying the notation) as:

$$R_x = \frac{N_x(2)}{N_{x-10}(1) - D \pm M} \quad (5.2)$$

The ratios for the population aged x and above at the time of the second census will be provided. For instance, the ratio at age 90 and above measures the actual population aged 90 and over (at the time of the second census) relative to its expected value based on the number enumerated in 1970 at ages 80 and over minus subsequent deaths and migrations to the open-ended cohort. The cumulation allows observation of the ratio trend while dampening error-induced extreme values at particular ages. It is insensitive to any errors of age reporting in deaths or population that occur within the population above the age that begins the open-ended age interval. The change in the size of the cohort as measured at two successive censuses ideally should be due to only mortality and migration. A ratio of 1.00 would indicate this ideal scenario. In fact, however, the reported count can be affected by (1) coverage errors in either or both censuses, (2) under- (or over-) enumeration in the death registration data and/or immigration statistics, and (3) characteristic (age, sex, race) misreporting in any or all of the data sources (Ewbank, 1981; Shryock and Siegel, 1976; Condran et al., 1991).

The ratio of observed to expected population is a useful diagnostic tool if patterns of deviation from 1.00 can be interpreted in terms of these underlying data errors. It is not highly precise, however, because different forms of error can produce the same patterns of ratios. Nonetheless, it can help to discriminate among competing alternatives.

HOW AGE OVERSTATEMENT AFFECTS THE RATIOS, BASED ON SIMULATION RESULTS

In order to evaluate the effects of varying patterns of age misstatement on the observed/expected ratios, Condran, Himes and Preston (1991) introduced simulated errors into data from the Netherlands that were constrained to have perfect consistency between two population age distributions and deaths. Age is assumed to be correctly reported until age 70. Beginning at age 70, however, four hypothesized patterns of age overstatement were introduced in the simulations:

Table 5.1		
Patterns of Age Misreporting, Based on Simulations		
Misre-porting Pattern	Proportion Misreporting Increases at Rate of:	Proportion of those Misreporting who Reported Older Ages:
1	0.01 at each age	Incr. from 0.3 to 0.7[1]
2	0.02 at each age	Incr. from 0.3 to 0.7[1]
3	0.01 at each age	Is 1.0 at every age
4	0.02 at each age	Is 1.0 at every age
Source: Condran et al.,1991, p.42. **Note:** [1] Increases with age.		

Results of three sets of simulations are presented. In the first set, the age overstatement patterns were limited to the two population age distributions. Figure 5.1 clearly demonstrates that age overstatement confined to the two population distributions results in a downward trend in the ratio series. To understand why the ratio declines below 1.00, refer to equation 5.2. An error in one component of the denominator (in this case, inflation of $N_{x-10}(1)$ by age overstatement) introduces disproportionate effects in the denominator. Even though the rapid tapering off in the age distribution can result in $N_x(2)$ being more inflated than $N_{x-10}(1)$, eventually the inflation of the denominator exceeds that of the numerator and the ratios fall.

In the second set of simulations, the same patterns of net age overstatement were introduced in both the censuses and in the death registration statistics. As shown in Figure 5.2, simulations with identical error in both sources produced increasing ratios. This important result is robust to the extent of error introduced (Condran et al., 1991). It reflects the fact that age distributions taper off more and more rapidly as age advances, so that the *same* percentage of

Figure 5.1

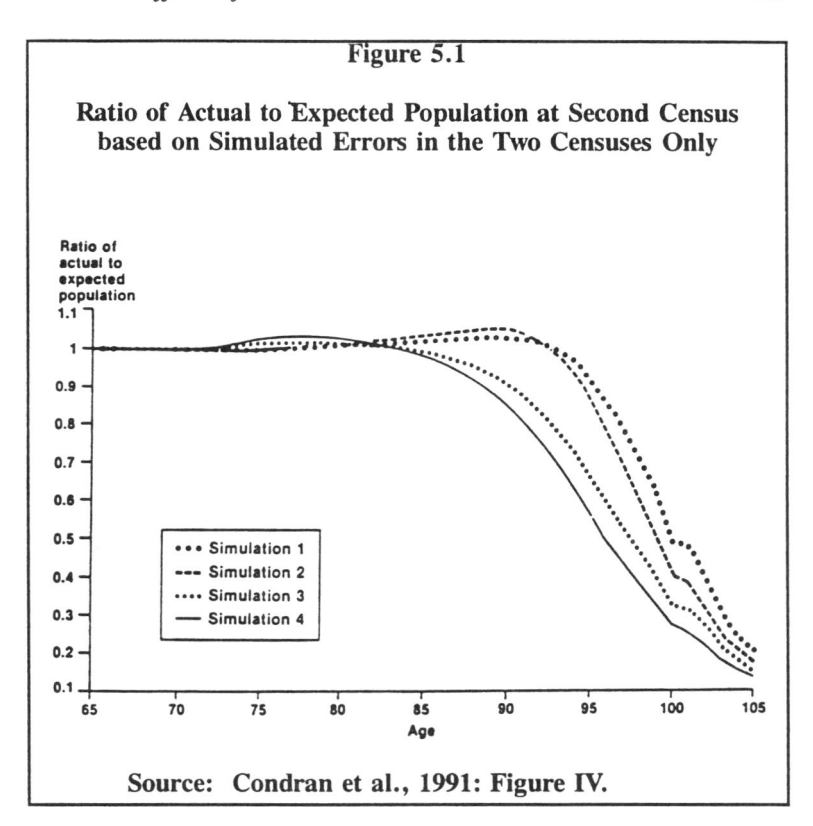

Ratio of Actual to Expected Population at Second Census based on Simulated Errors in the Two Censuses Only

Source: Condran et al., 1991: Figure IV.

persons who overstate their true age will introduce larger *percentage* errors in the reported age distributions at the very advanced ages. That is, $N_x(2)$ has a larger inflation factor than $N_{x-10}(1)$. In this case, some of the inflation in $N_{x-10}(1)$ is offset in its effects on the denominator by an inflation in D.

In a third simulation, Condran et al. (*ibid*) demonstrated that when deaths had either no error or a substantially lower level of error than the censuses, the ratios of actual to expected population declined with age to values well below unity. This pattern is illustrated by Figure 5.3.

110   Racial Differences in Life Expectancy

Figure 5.2

Ratio of Actual to Expected Population at the Second Census based on Simulated Errors in the Two Censuses and in the Death Registration Data

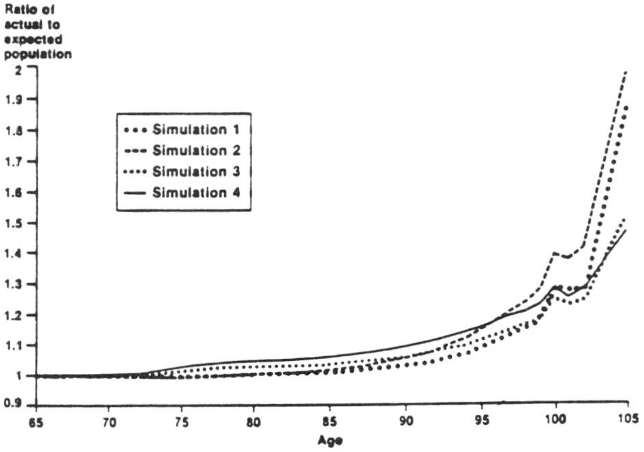

Source: Condran, et al., 1991: Figure V.

Figure 5.3

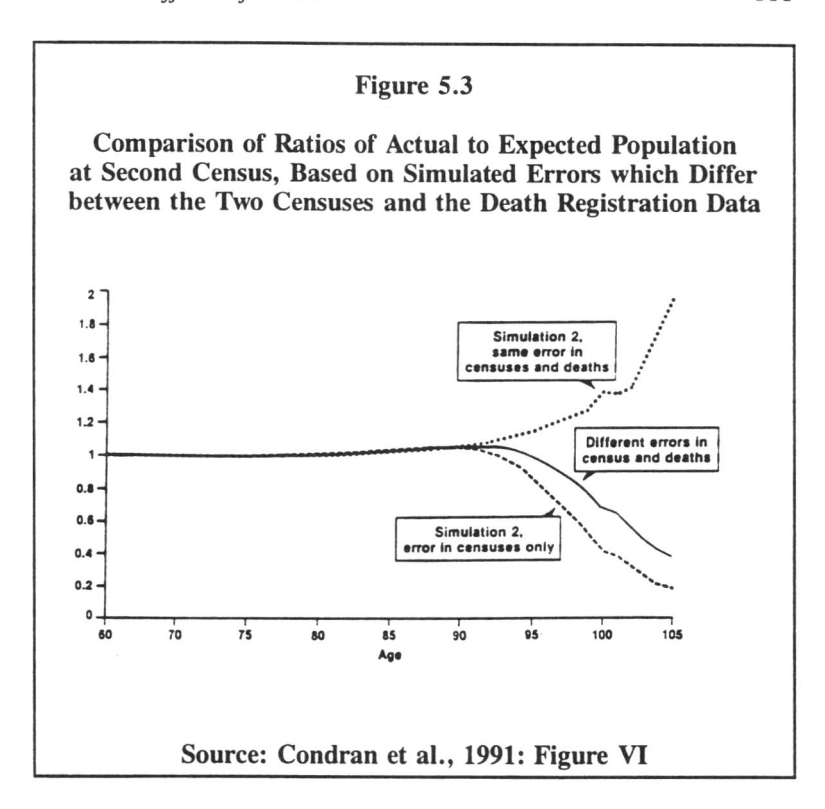

Comparison of Ratios of Actual to Expected Population at Second Census, Based on Simulated Errors which Differ between the Two Censuses and the Death Registration Data

Source: Condran et al., 1991: Figure VI

DERIVING ESTIMATES OF THE "TRUE" 1980 AND 1990 POPULATION AGE DISTRIBUTIONS AND INTERCENSAL DEATHS

Expanding upon the work of Condran et al. (1991), the following sections describe the effects of introducing simulated errors into a "perfect" data set typical of the current demographic conditions of the United States. The first section describes the methodology employed to derive the "true" US population and death distributions in the 1980 to 1990 intercensal period. The second section considers the effect of simulated coverage errors in the data sources on the intercensal ratios. Finally, the effects of three types of age reporting patterns on the ratios are considered: accurate reporting, age overstatement, and age understatement. These sections differ from the work of Condran et al. (*ibid*) in two important respects. First, while Condran et al. considered the effects of age misreporting, we expand the analyses to all of the major sources of error observed in census and vital registration data. Second, we use baseline data from the United States for the analyses while the work of Condran et al. was based on data from the Netherlands.

The Methodology

The modelling methodology is based on forward survival of the "true" (without error) 1980 baseline population to its correct level in 1990. As shown in Chapter 2, however, the empirically-derived enumerations of the 1980 age distribution are biased by both coverage and age misreporting errors. The following sections describe a methodology which allows approximation of the true US 1980 age distribution in the absence of error. The "true" 1980 age distribution is then used as the basis for calculation of the "true" number of intercensal deaths and the "true" 1990 population age distribution. Finally, calculated values for the simulated 1980 and 1990 populations and intercensal deaths in the absence of error are presented.

Estimating the simulated 1980 "true" age distribution

In any population closed to migration, the number of persons aged x at a point in time, denoted by $N(x)$, can be calculated by:

$$N(x) = N(a) \cdot {}_{x-a}P_a \ e^{\int_a^x r(u)du} \qquad (5.3)$$

where $N(a)$ is the number of persons aged a, ${}_{x-a}P_a$ is the probability of surviving from age a to age x according to the period mortality rates, and $r(u)$ is the growth rate of the population aged u at the point in time (Bennett and Horiuchi, 1981).

As noted by Preston and Bennett (1983), the ratio of populations at the moment in time can be expressed completely in terms of age-specific mortality rates and growth rates between those ages. In elaborations of the model, Preston and Bennett (*ibid*) showed that the closed population's age structure can be converted into that of a corresponding stationary population subject to the same mortality conditions (Bennett and Horiuchi, 1984). In discrete terms, approximated for five-year age groups, the equation developed by Preston and Bennett is:

$$_5L_y = {_5N_y}\, e^{R(x)}, \quad \text{where} \quad (5.4)$$

$$R(x) = 5 \sum_{0}^{y-5} {_5r_x} + 2.5\, {_5r_y} \quad (5.5)$$

The number of person years lived in a five-year interval in a stationary population is calculated by multiplying the number of persons (aged y to y+5) in the population by e raised to the cumulated growth rate.

Our application of the procedure required two minor adjustments. First, our conversion is in the opposite direction, i.e. a life table is utilized to estimate the simulated 1980 US white male age distribution. Second, the equations were modified to allow estimation of the simulated population's age distribution by single years of age.

$$_1N_y = {_1L_y}\, e^{R(x)}, \quad \text{where} \quad (5.6)$$

$$R(x) = \sum_{o}^{y-1} {_1r_x} + 0.5\, {_1r_y} \quad (5.7)$$

To implement Equation (5.6), $_1L_y$ values were utilized from the official 1980 US white male life table (National Center for Health Statistics, 1985). The age-specific growth rates are calculated from the empirical 1980 and 1990 race-modified white male census counts by single years of age:

$$_1r_x = \frac{\ln \dfrac{_1N_x\,(1980)}{_1N_x\,(1990)}}{10} \quad (5.8)$$

Because of irregularities in the calculated growth rates at the oldest ages, it was assumed that $_1r_x$ for $x \geq 100$ equalled .0250, an intermediate value within the range of .0249 and .0257 as calculated for ages 96 to 98.

The advantages of use of the Preston-Bennett procedure to estimate the age distribution of the simulated 1980 population include: (1) relative insensitivity to age misstatement at the older ages, (2) lack of required assumption of population stability, (3) availability of empirical input data by single years of age, sex, and race, and, (4) ease of application (Preston and Bennett, 1983; United Nations, 1983).

A disadvantage is that the method assumes that the population is closed to migration. Note, however, that the impact of the violation in the aged US population is likely to be minimal given the relative importance of attrition from mortality relative to the impact of net immigration (see Chapter 3). A second disadvantage is that errors in the input data (the estimated growth rates or the life table $_1L_y$ values) could introduce bias.

Estimating the simulated "true" 1990 age distribution

The simulated 1990 population is estimated by the forward survival of the 1980 simulated "true" baseline population using official 1980 life table ($_1L_x$) values:

$$_1N_x (1990) = {_1N_{x-10}^{(1980)}} * \frac{_1L_x}{_1L_{x-10}} \qquad (5.9)$$

where $_1L_x/_1L_{x-10}$ represents the proportion of the population aged x-10 in 1980 who survive to age x in 1990.

For example, the population aged 70 in 1990 ($_1N_{70}$ (1990)) is calculated by multiplying the population aged 60 in 1980 ($_1N_{60}$ (1980)) by the survival ratio $_1L_{80}/_1L_{70}$.

Estimating the simulated intercensal distribution of deaths

The difference between the 1980 and 1990 simulated age distributions provides an intercensal estimate of the number of deaths for each birth cohort. The ten year estimate of deaths is then converted into an array of deaths by single years of age and single calendar years, again using techniques of forward survival and applying separation factors.

The computational procedure to calculate deaths in a single calendar year involves a number of steps, described below for the year

1980. First, single year survivorship ratios, which describe the probability of surviving from 1980 (at age x, in completed years) to 1981 (at age x+1) are calculated using the 1980 life table $_1L_x$ values. For instance, the equation to determine the survivorship probability between ages 60 and 61 is:

$$_1S_{60,61} = \frac{_1L_{61}}{_1L_{60}} \quad (5.10)$$

Second, the number of survivors in the one year period between 1980 and 1981 is calculated by multiplying $_1N_x$ by the survival ratio is step 1. For instance, the number of survivors to age 61 in 1981 is calculated by multiplying the number aged 60 in 1980 by the survivorship ratio in step 1:

$$_1N_{61} = {_1N_{60}} * \frac{_1L_{61}}{_1L_{60}} \quad (5.11)$$

Third, the difference between the number aged x+1 in 1981 (survivors) and the number aged x in 1980 represents the number of deaths to that cohort in the one year time frame:

$$_1D_{60} = {_1N_{60}^{(1980)}} - {_1N_{61}^{(1981)}} \quad (5.12)$$

Alternatively, the number of deaths can be calculated directly (omitting step 2) by the following equation:

$$_1D_{60} = {_1N_{60}^{(1980)}} * (1 - \frac{_1L_{61}}{_1L_{60}}) \quad (5.13)$$

Finally, it is noted that deaths to the cohort aged 60 (in completed years) in calendar year 1980 occur both at exact age 60 and at exact age 61. We assume that half occur at each age.

The process is repeated for each subsequent calendar year by surviving the most recent year's population forward one year.

Estimates of the "true" number of persons and deaths in the simulated population.

Table 5.2 presents the results of the simulations described above. By construction, consistency between the reported intercensal changes in the size of cohorts and the number of intervening deaths is maintained throughout the age range in the "true" simulations. At each age, the ratio of the actual to the expected population in 1990, calculated on the basis of equation 12, will equal 1.00.

$$R = ratio\ of\ \frac{actual\ population\ (1990)}{expected\ population\ (1990)}$$

$$= \frac{actual\ population\ (1990)}{baseline\ population\ (1980) - intercensal\ deaths} \quad (5.14)$$

For example, the following values (cumulated from Table 5.2) for the population aged 85 and above in 1980 were calculated: the baseline population in 1980 equalled 39,576, the number of intercensal deaths was 36,708 and the actual population in 1990 was found to be 2,868. The ratio of actual population (2,868) to expected population (39,576-36,708) was unity.

Table 5.2
Estimates of the "True" Simulated Populations and the Intercensal Number of Deaths in the Absence of Coverage Error or Age Misreporting

Age in 1980 (A)	Population in 1980 (B)	Intercensal Deaths (C)	Population in 1990 (D=B-C)
40	86,322	3,747	82,575
41	82,701	3,960	78,741
42	79,401	4,189	75,212
43	76,321	4,432	71,890
44	71,804	4,588	67,217
45	67,237	4,722	62,515
46	65,582	5,056	60,526
47	63,801	5,387	58,414
48	61,072	5,639	55,432
49	58,403	5,887	52,516
50	56,987	6,266	50,720
51	55,869	6,698	49,171
52	55,168	7,206	47,961
53	54,471	7,749	46,722
54	54,261	8,394	45,867
55	53,823	9,100	45,070
56	53,823	9,800	44,022
57	53,730	10,589	43,141
58	53,727	11,443	42,284
59	53,700	12,344	41,356

Age in 1980	Popln (1980)	Deaths	Popln (1990)
60	54,057	13,395	40,661
61	53,362	14,238	39,124
62	52,490	15,058	37,431
63	51,440	15,836	35,604
64	49,973	16,475	33,498
65	48,360	17,038	31,322
66	46,654	17,536	29,118
67	44,808	17,942	26,866
68	42,899	18,271	24,629
69	40,943	18,515	22,428
70	38,631	18,518	20,113
71	36,209	18,371	17,839
72	33,986	18,224	15,762
73	31,759	17,970	13,789
74	29,570	17,620	11,950
75	27,367	17,138	10,229
76	25,130	16,502	8,628
77	22,832	15,683	7,149
78	20,700	14,830	5,870
79	18,484	13,768	4,717
80	16,306	12,586	3,720
81	14,492	11,558	2,934
82	12,665	10,409	2,257
83	10,893	9,201	1,692
84	9,252	8,013	1,239

Table 5.2 (continued)			
Age in 1980	Popln (1980)	Deaths	Popln (1990)
85	7,839	6,943	896
86	6,579	5,943	637
87	5,444	5,001	443
88	4,470	4,165	305
89	3,641	3,435	207
90	2,882	2,745	136
91	2,244	2,156	88
92	1,755	1,698	58
93	1,358	1,321	37
94	1,013	990	24
95	735	720	15
96	523	514	9
97	366	361	5
98	251	248	3
99	170	168	2
100+	305	302	3
85+	39,576	36,708	2,868

Source: Derived from simulations.

Notes: (1) Rows can be read horizontally; (2) Age refers to age in completed years in 1980; (3) Population in 1990 = Baseline population in 1980-intercensal deaths; (4) Small deviations are due to rounding.

With introduction of error into any of the three components of the equation, deviation away from unity is expected. The following sections describe the effect of various coverage and age misreporting errors on the ratios. The "true" set of simulations will provide the error-free basis for comparison.

Simulations with Introduced Coverage Errors

We computed three sets of simulations that demonstrate the effects of various combinations of coverage error in the censuses and death registration (see Table 5.3). Reiterating, coverage error refers to the degree to which the enumerated population or the number of deaths differs from the true number. Introduction of content errors, or misreporting of characteristics, will be considered later. The three simulated patterns represent various combinations of three different levels of coverage in the censuses and death registration system: (1) complete coverage, (2) net over-enumeration, and, (3) net under-enumeration (or under-registration). In all three sets of simulations, it was assumed that coverage was complete up to age 60. At that age and beyond, the proportion inaccurate (in those simulations which assume error) at each age was held constant at five percent.

As seen in Table 5.3 (last column), various combinations of coverage completeness in the census and death enumerations produced similar results, with the most prevalence pattern being a declining ratio series. A summary of the implications of these simulations will be presented later.

Table 5.3
Simulations with Introduced Coverage Error

First Census Coverage	Second Census Coverage	Death Registration Coverage	Pattern	Simulation Result: Ratios Pattern
Accurate	Accurate	Accurate	AAA	Straight Line (at 1.00)
Accurate	Accurate	Under-Registration	AAU	Declining
Accurate	Overcount	Accurate	AOA	Straight Line (at 1.05)
Accurate	Overcount	Under-Registration	AOU	Declining
Accurate	Undercount	Accurate	AUA	Straight Line (at 0.95)
Accurate	Undercount	Under-Registration	AUU	Declining
Overcount	Accurate	Accurate	OAA	Declining
Overcount	Accurate	Under-Registration	OAU	Declining
Overcount	Overcount	Accurate	OOA	Declining
Overcount	Overcount	Under-Registration	OOU	Declining
Overcount	Undercount	Accurate	OUA	Declining
Overcount	Undercount	Under-Registration	OUU	Declining

Table 5.3 (continued)

First Census Coverage	Second Census Coverage	Death Registration Coverage	Pattern	Simulation Result: Ratios Pattern
Undercount	Accurate	Accurate	UAA	Increasing
Undercount	Accurate	Under-Registration	UAU	Declining
Undercount	Overcount	Accurate	UOA	Increasing
Undercount	Overcount	Under-Registration	UOU	Declining
Undercount	Undercount	Accurate	UUA	Increasing
Undercount	Undercount	Under-Registration	UUU	Declining

Note: We do not simulate the highly unrealistic case of over-registration of deaths. Note, however, that the pattern AAO is equivalent to UUA.

In summary, the following major possibilities for coverage error and their implications for the age-pattern of ratios of observed to expected population can be distinguished, assuming no age misreporting:

1. If $N_{x-10}(1)$ is overcounted relative to its true level, any combination of coverage error in $N_x(2)$ and D will produce declining ratios. The only exception is the combination OOO, which means that all three sources are overcounted to the same extent. With pattern OOO, increases in the ratio series are observed.

2. If $N_{x-10}(1)$ is undercounted relative to its true level, the age pattern of the ratios depends on relative coverage in the death registration system. If D is accurately reported, implying that coverage in deaths is better than in the first census, the ratio series will increase. If deaths are also undercounted (N_{x-10} coverage equals that of D), then the ratios will decline with age.

3. If $N_{x-10}(1)$ is accurately reported, the pattern of the ratios again depends upon coverage in the death registration system. If deaths are also accurately reported, then the age pattern of the ratios will be constant with age and its level will be the relative completeness of $N_x(2)$. If deaths are underregistered, implying that coverage is better in the first census, a declining series is observed regardless of the relative completeness of $N_x(2)$.

Furthermore, simulations suggested that, in the event of either *no* content error or *less* content error in deaths relative to both censuses, the age-pattern of the ratios is similar, differing only in the magnitude of the ratios at individual ages and in the age at which rapid movement away from unity begins. With the *same* error in both deaths and in the censuses, however, a reversal in the age-pattern of the ratios is observed.

Simulations with Introduced Age Misreporting Errors

Referring to Table 5.4, six sets of simulations that demonstrate the effects of various combinations of age misreporting on R(x) were carried out. Simulated patterns of age reporting, introduced in both the censuses and the death registration statistics, consider: (1) consistent reporting of age, (2) net overstatement of age, in which a larger percentage of persons report themselves to be older than their true ages, and, (3) net understatement of age, in which persons are reported younger than their true ages.

We also considered a pattern of normalized symmetric misreporting in which an equal proportion overstate and understate their ages. For the five percent of an age category assumed to misreport age, the difference between reported age and true age was hypothesized to approximate a normal distribution of errors. With an assumed standard deviation of 1.5 years for those misreporting, about 99% will either overstate or understate their correct age within 4.5 years. The miniscule remaining proportion (1%) was allocated based on the entire population age distribution, which allowed for misreporting to *any* age. Because the symmetric misreporting pattern is almost indisguishable from the "accurate" pattern in the simulation results, we exclude the symmetric results from this presentation.

In the simulations which allow misreporting, it was assumed that age was accurately reported until age 60. (Note that Condran et al. (1991) introduce error beginning at age 70. We allow error beginning as early as age 60 because of the possibility of age misreporting in age range 60 up to 70 in the United States, particularly for the African American population). Beyond age 60, the proportion misreporting at each age was held constant at five percent. Inthe cases of overstatement and understatement, of those who misrepresent their true age, 5/15 are assumed to misreport by one year, 4/15 by two years, 3/15 by three years, 2/15 by four years, and 1/15 by five years. No deviations greater than five years were introduced. While age misstatement was first introduced at age 60, this procedure allowed individuals corrected aged 60-64 to report back into the 55-59 age group.

Again, the principal output of the simulations is the ratio of actual population to expected population at age x and above at the time of the second census.

Table 5.4
Simulations with Various Patterns of Age Misreporting

Age Reporting Pattern in:			Pattern	Simulation Result: Ratios Pattern
First Census	**Second Census**	**Death Registration**		
Accurate	Accurate	Accurate	AAA	Straight Line
Accurate	Accurate	Overstated	AAO	Increasing
Accurate	Accurate	Understated	AAU	Declining
Accurate	Overstated	Accurate	AOA	Increasing
Accurate	Overstated	Overstated	AOO	Declining
Accurate	Overstated	Understated	AOU	Increasing
Accurate	Understated	Accurate	AUA	Declining
Accurate	Understated	Overstated	AUO	Declining
Accurate	Understated	Understated	AUU	Increasing

Table 5.4 (continued)
Simulations with Various Patterns of Age Misreporting

Age Reporting Pattern in:			Pattern	Simulation Result: Ratios Pattern
First Census	Second Census	Death Registration		
Overstated	Accurate	Accurate	OAA	Declining
Overstated	Overstated	Accurate	OOA	Declining
Overstated	Understated	Accurate	OUA	Declining
Overstated	Accurate	Overstated	OAO	Increasing
Overstated	Overstated	Overstated	OOO	Increasing
Overstated	Understated	Overstated	OUO	Increasing
Overstated	Accurate	Understated	OAU	Declining
Overstated	Overstated	Understated	OOU	Declining
Overstated	Understated	Understated	OUU	Declining

Table 5.4 (continued)
Simulations with Various Patterns of Age Misreporting

Age Reporting Pattern in:				Simulation Result: Ratios Pattern
First Census	Second Census	Death Registration	Pattern	
Understated	Accurate	Accurate	UAA	Increasing
Understated	Overstated	Accurate	UOA	Increasing
Understated	Understated	Accurate	UUA	Increasing
Understated	Accurate	Overstated	UAO	Increasing
Understated	Overstated	Overstated	UOO	Increasing
Understated	Understated	Overstated	UUO	Increasing
Understated	Accurate	Understated	UAU	Declining
Understated	Overstated	Understated	UOU	Declining
Understated	Understated	Understated	UUU	Declining

Summarizing the effects of various age reporting patterns on the intercensal ratios of observed to expected population:

1. *If age reporting in the first census is overstated and:*

(a) Age reporting in the death registration is overstated, then an increasing ratio series is observed, regardless of pattern in second census.

(b) Age reporting in the death registration is accurate or understated, then a declining ratio series is observed, regardless of pattern in the second census.

2. *If age reporting in the first census is understated and:*

(a) Age reporting in the death registration is understated, then a declining ratio series is observed, regardless of the pattern in second census.

(b) Age reporting in the death registration is accurate or overstated, then an increasing ratio series is observed, regardless of pattern in second census.

3. *If age in the first census is accurate and:*

(a) Age reporting in the death registration is overstated, then a declining ratio series is observed, regardless of pattern in second census.

(b) Age reporting in the death registration is understated, then an increasing ratio series is observed, regardless of pattern in the second census.

(c) Age reporting in the death registration is accurate, then it depends on the pattern of age reporting in the second census:

>(c.1) If age is understated in the second census, then a declining ratio series is observed.

>(c.2) If age is overstated in the second census, then an increasing ratio series is observed.

Simulations further suggested that, in the event of either *no misreporting error* or *less misreporting of age* in deaths relative to both censuses, the age-pattern of the ratios is similar, differing only in the magnitudes of the ratios at individual ages and in the age at which rapid movement away from unity begins. With the *same level of misreporting* in both deaths and in the censuses, however, a reversal in the age-pattern of the ratios is observed.

A final issue is the effect of our modelling assumption that the proportion misreporting at each age at 60 and above is *constant* at five percent. To test the sensitivity of the simplistic assumption, sensitivity analyses were carried out in which we assumed an increasing proportion misreport with age. In all cases, the ratio patterns remained identical to that observed with constant misreporting. The effect of the increasing proportion misreporting assumption was to accelerate the timing of the deviation away from unity in the ratio series.

VI

US Results: Errors in the Ratios and their Effects on Life Expectancy

The previous sections presented results of simulations that were carried out in order to evaluate the potential effects of plausible content and coverage errors in censuses and death registration on intercensal ratios of observed to expected population. The simulations extend earlier work by Condran et al. (1991) who evaluated the effects of age overstatement on the population ratios. This research has confirmed the work of Condran et al. (*ibid*) on age overstatement using a dataset from the United States, and has expanded research in this area to consider other patterns of age misreporting as well as coverage error.

The following possibilities for coverage error (assuming no age misreporting) were identified and their implications for the age-pattern of ratios of observed/expected population were distinguished:

1. If the first census is *over*counted relative to its true level, any combination of coverage error in the second census and death registration will produce declining ratios. The only exception is the combination in which all three sources are overcounted to the same extent. With this pattern, increases in the ratio series are observed.

2. If the first census is *under*counted relative to its true level, the age pattern of the ratios depends on relative coverage in the death registration system. If deaths are accurately reported, implying that coverage in deaths is better than in the first census, the ratio series will increase. If deaths are also undercounted (N_{x-10} coverage equals that of D), then the ratios will decline with age.

3. If the first census is accurately reported, the pattern of the ratios again depends upon coverage in the death registration system. If deaths are also accurately reported, then the age pattern of the ratios will be constant with age and its level will be the relative completeness of the second census. If deaths are underregistered, implying that coverage is better in the first census, a declining series is observed regardless of the relative completeness of the second census.

Furthermore, simulations suggested that, in the event of either *no* content error or *less* content error in deaths relative to both censuses, the age-pattern of the ratios is similar, differing only in the magnitude of the ratios at individual ages and in the age at which rapid movement away from unity begins. With the *same* error in both deaths and in the censuses, however, a reversal in the age-pattern of the ratios is observed.

The effects of various major age reporting patterns on the intercensal ratios of observed to expected population were also considered. In summary, the results were:

1. *If age reporting in the first census is overstated and:*

(a) Age reporting in the death registration is overstated, then an increasing ratio series is observed, regardless of pattern in second census.

(b) Age reporting in the death registration is accurate or understated, then a declining ratio series is observed, regardless of pattern in the second census.

2. *If age reporting in the first census is understated and:*

(a) Age reporting in the death registration is understated, then a declining ratio series is observed, regardless of the pattern in second census.

(b) Age reporting in the death registration is accurate or overstated, then an increasing ratio series is observed, regardless of pattern in second census.

3. *If age in the first census is accurate and:*

(a) Age reporting in the death registration is overstated, then a declining ratio series is observed, regardless of pattern in second census.

(b) Age reporting in the death registration is understated, then an increasing ratio series is observed, regardless of pattern in the second census.

(c) Age reporting in the death registration is accurate, then it depends on the pattern of age reporting in the second census:

> (c.1) If age is understated in the second census, then a declining ratio series is observed.

> (c.2) If age is overstated in the second census, then an increasing ratio series is observed.

Simulations further suggested that, in the event of either *no misreporting error* or *less misreporting of age* in deaths relative to both censuses, the age-pattern of the ratios is similar, differing only in the magnitudes of the ratios at individual ages and in the age at which rapid movement away from unity begins. With the *same level of misreporting* in both deaths and in the censuses, however, a reversal in the age-pattern of the ratios is observed.

A final issue was the effect of our modelling assumption that the proportion misreporting at each age at 60 and above is *constant* at five percent. To test the sensitivity of the simplistic assumption, sensitivity analyses were carried out in which we assumed an increasing proportion misreport with age. In all cases, the ratio patterns remained identical to that observed with constant misreporting. The effect of the increasing proportion misreporting assumption was to accelerate the timing of the deviation away from unity in the ratio series.

While these simulations have provided useful insight into the combinations of error that can produce inconsistencies in empirically-derived ratios of observed to expected populations, they are not intended to be all-inclusive. For instance, an interesting issue not addressed in these simulations is the effect on the ratios of various combinations of *both* content and coverage errors in each of the basic data sources.

The fundamental task in this final chapter is to identify and evaluate inconsistencies and inadequacies found in the US data sources at the oldest ages for four sex-race combinations: white males, white females, black males, and black females. Results will be presented separately for the 1970-1980 and the 1980-1990 intercensal periods. Heavy reliance will be placed on the use of cohort analysis to evaluate the quality of old age statistics. The degree of consistency between reported intercensal changes in the size of cohorts and the number of intervening deaths and net migration will be measured. The methodology, which has not been previously used to study age misreporting patterns in old age in the US, will be diagnostic in nature, highlighting data inconsistencies in the intercensal experience of the cohorts. The principal output will be age-specific ratios of the enumerated population to the expected population for each of the four sex-race groups.

DATA INCONSISTENCIES IN THE OLD-AGE US POPULATIONS

In the following sections, empirically-based ratios for the US white and African American old age populations will be examined in light of both the simulation results and evidence in the literature regarding the nature of coverage and content errors in the censuses and death registration statistics.

Intercensal cohort analysis was carried out for the four sex-race groups in the United States in the 1970-1980 and 1980-1990 periods. Table 6.1 presents the calculated ratios of the observed to expected population above various ages in the United States by race, sex, and intercensal period.

Within race categories for a particular time period, the male and female ratio series follow very similar patterns, differing only in magnitude. In all cases, the degree of inconsistency increases with age, although any systematic and significant departure from 1.00 is postponed until age 95 and beyond for whites in 1980-1990.

Table 6.1
Ratio of Observed to Expected Population Above Age X at Second Census based on Intercensal Cohort Methodology: United States, by Race, Sex, and Intercensal Period

Age (x)	1970 to 1980 Whites M	Whites F	Blacks M	Blacks F	1980 to 1990 Whites M	Whites F	Blacks M	Blacks F
50	1.030	1.028	1.090	1.053	0.998	0.999	1.019	0.985
55	1.034	1.031	1.100	1.062	0.999	1.000	1.018	0.986
60	1.035	1.032	1.106	1.067	0.998	1.000	1.011	0.983
65	1.042	1.040	1.110	1.073	0.997	1.001	0.999	0.980
70	1.038	1.036	1.058	1.024	0.993	0.999	0.956	0.951
75	1.043	1.038	0.972	0.966	0.989	0.997	0.903	0.914
80	1.041	1.045	0.887	0.925	0.985	0.998	0.833	0.874
85	1.100	1.103	0.810	0.907	0.971	0.997	0.728	0.801
90	1.125	1.149	0.716	0.844	0.931	1.007	0.579	0.692
95	1.071	1.199	0.693	0.840	0.794	1.014	0.438	0.554
100	0.614	0.937	1.022	1.253	0.275	0.560	0.253	0.336

RESULTS FOR WHITES

Whites in the 1970-80 Intercensal Period

Figure 6.1 presents the ratios of observed population to the expected population at age x for the white male and female populations in the 1970-1980 intercensal period. The actual population (in 1980) generally surpassed the expected level, but fell within five percent of unity for most single years of age between 61 and about 80. Increasing divergence away from unity is observed for the duration of the series. An exception to the pattern is observed at exact ages 50, 60, 70, 80, and 90. Whereas at all other ages the ratios surpassed unity, the calculated ratio of actual to expected population at these ages fell short of unity, indicating that the actual population in 1980 is less than expected based on the 1970 population and subsequent deaths and migration. Significant declines in the ratios are also observed at exact ages 95 and 98 although the actual population in 1980 continues to surpass its expected value at these ages.

Figure 6.1

Whites, by Sex, 1970-80
Ratio: Observed to Expected Population

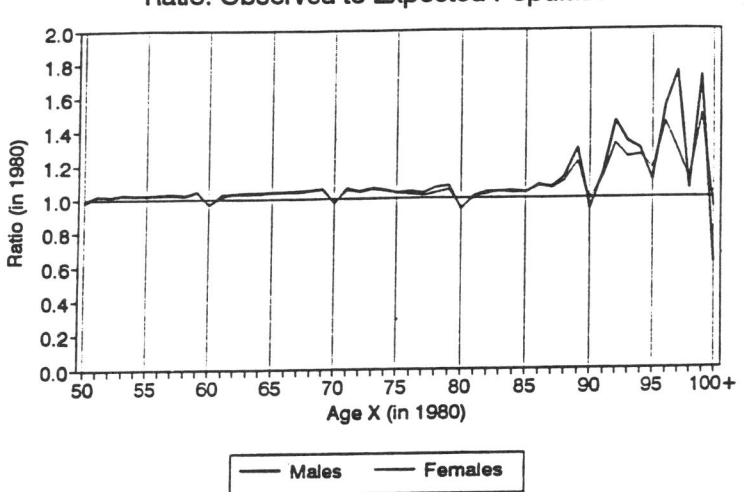

Because less coverage error exists in the 1980 census relative to 1970 (US Bureau of the Census, 1988), our first instinct was to attribute the plunges in the ratio series to more pronounced age heaping in the 1970 census enumerations on the terminal -0 ages relative to digit heaping on those ages in the 1980 census. This interpretation, however, contradicts evaluation results published in a Census Bureau publication (1983a). That study suggested that age heaping in the 1970 and 1980 censuses was diminished to such low levels that it was indistinguishable from other errors in the data from real fluctuations due to past variations in births, deaths, and net migration. Replicating the methodology employed by the Census Bureau, we used Myers' Blended Method (1940) to evaluate the extent of reporting preference for ages ending in particular digits. We limit our analysis to white males aged 50 up to age 90 in the 1970 and 1980 censuses. Because age misreporting generally increases with age, limitation of the calculations to the older population can be expected to result in more age misreporting than observed in Census Bureau estimates which were based on the age distribution of the entire population. Referring to Table 6.2, very low levels of age misreporting are observed at each terminal age, confirming the analysis by the Census Bureau. Results from the Myers' Method indicate the extent of concentration or avoidance of a particular terminal digit. In the absence of error, about ten percent of the population will have terminal digit -0; ten percent will have terminal digit -1; and so forth. The actual percent distribution and absolute deviation from ten percent is presented in the table.

The summary index, which measures the minimum proportion of persons in the population for whom an age with an incorrect final digit is recorded (Shryock and Siegel, 1976), measured only 0.75 for the white male population aged 50 to 89 in 1970. The 1980 population, which we speculated might have better reporting of age, actually had a *higher* summary index (0.83) of age heaping, although it remained very low. Seven terminal ages (except 4, 5, 8) had worse heaping in 1980 relative to 1970.

Our next step was to ascertain the degree of terminal digit preference in the registered deaths in the 1970-1980 intercensal period. Again, we found very low levels of digit preference in the source, with a summary index equal to 0.78. These results are also presented in Table 6.2.

Table 6.2
Calculation of a Preference Index for Terminal Digits by Myers' Blended Method for US White Males Aged 50-89 in the 1970-1980 Intercensal Period

Terminal Digit X		Blended 1970 Census	Blended 1980 Census	Blended Deaths
0	Percent Distrib.	10.26	9.73	9.72
	Over/Under Expected?	Over	Under	Under
1	Percent Distrib.	9.83	9.73	9.80
	Over/Under Expected?	Under	Under	Under
2	Percent Distrib.	9.91	9.85	9.83
	Over/Under Expected?	Under	Under	Under
3	Percent Distrib.	9.87	9.82	9.86
	Over/Under Expected?	Under	Under	Under
4	Percent Distrib.	10.09	10.02	10.03
	Over/Under Expected?	Over	Over	Over
5	Percent Distrib.	10.18	10.15	10.09
	Over/Under Expected?	Over	Over	Over
6	Percent Distrib.	10.11	10.12	10.15
	Over/Under Expected?	Over	Over	Over
7	Percent Distrib.	10.11	10.15	10.17
	Over/Under Expected?	Over	Over	Over
8	Percent Distrib.	10.21	10.20	10.05
	Over/Under Expected?	Over	Over	Over
9	Percent Distrib.	9.86	10.23	10.28
	Over/Under Expected?	Under	Over	Over
Summary Index of Prefer.		0.76	0.83	0.78

Source: Adapted from: Myers, R.J. 1940. Errors and bias in the reporting of ages in census data. *Transactions of the Actuarial Society of America*, 41, part 2(104):413.
Notes: (1) "% distribution": proportion of total population reporting on the terminal digit; (2) "summary index of age preference" for all terminal digits: 1/2 the sum of absolute deviations from 10%. If age heaping is nonexistent, index would be zero. The index is an estimate of the minimum proportion of persons in the pop. for whom an age with an incorrect final digit is reported (Shryock and Siegel, 1976).

Based on calculations using Myers' Blended Method, the following generalizations can be made about age heaping in the white male population aged 50 to 89 in the 1970 to 1980 intercensal period:

1. Very low levels of digit preference exist in the two decennial censuses (1970 and 1980) and in death registration statistics.

2. The number of persons reported with terminal digits 1, 2, and 3 was less than that expected in all three sources.

3. The number of persons reported with terminal digits 4, 5, 6, 7 and 8 was more than the expected value in all three sources.

4. Inconsistent patterns are realized at terminal digits 0 and 9. Reporting with terminal digit 0 was overestimated in 1970, while underreporting was observed in both the 1980 census and in deaths. In contrast, at terminal digit 9, underreporting was found in 1970 while overreporting was detected in 1980 and in deaths. There is no obvious explanation for the change in digit preference between the 1970 and the 1980 censuses. Respondents in both census years were requested to provide their month and year of birth in FOSDIC-readable form on the census questionnaire. Data on age was calculated by the computer by subtracting the date of birth from the census date.

While only low levels of age heaping were detected in all three sources, the errors discerned at terminal age -0 are cumulative on the ratios of observed to expected population. With overreporting into -0 in the 1970 census combined with underreporting in the 1980 census, the ratio will be less than that expected in the absence of age heaping. We can relate age -0 heaping to a simulation which has an overcount in the 1970 census, an undercount in the 1980 census and accurate deaths. The resultant pattern of age ratios is one in which the ratio is less than that expected in the absence of error. The heaping pattern in deaths is irrelevant. As shown in Chapter 5, regardless of whether deaths are accurate or undercounted, net overcount in the first census will result in a declining ratios series. Furthermore, while a pattern of age heaping is observed in deaths in a given year, each intercensal cohort passes through each digit in the ten years between 1970 and 1980. Similarly, troughs in the age pattern of the ratios are observed for whites at ages ending in -0 because too many individuals are reported with ages ending in -0 in 1970 while too few are reported in the 1980 census.

The ratio for the white centenarian populations was only 0.6141 for males and 0.9370 for females. These ratios indicate that the centenarian population in 1980 was less than its expected value based on the size of the 1970 population aged 90 and above and intercensal deaths. This result is unexpected based on evidence on the nature of error in our data sources. First, the white centenarian populations in 1970 in Census Bureau's unpublished tabulations appear to be undercounted, which would suggest ratios which *surpass* unity in 1980, ceteris paribus. Because of a large overcount in the official counts, the Census Bureau estimated the centenarian population in the unpublished tabulations by forward survival of the 1960 population using 1959-61 life table rates. Because the mortality rates used to close out the life tables were based on the experience of Civil War veterans, Siegel and Passel (1976) suggest that the survival rates of the extreme aged may have increased. With improvements in medical technology and care for the aged, the 1959-61 life tables may over-estimate mortality causing too few individuals to be estimated as centenarians in the 1970 census. Second, the US Bureau of the Census (1987b) argues that the 1980 centenarian population is overcounted, perhaps by as much as 25%, due to allocation procedures used by the US Bureau of the Census. Again, all these being equal, an overcount in the second census would suggest ratio values in 1980 which exceed unity.

Simulations presented in the previous chapter demonstrated that the combination of undercounted centenarian population in 1970, overcounted centenarian population in 1980, and accurate deaths would produce *increases* in the ratio of observed to expected population. In order to show the decrease observed in the empirically-based ratio for the centenarian population, under-registration in centenarian deaths is required. While the UOU coverage combination produces the required ratio, it is not conclusive evidence that the deaths are under-registered. The reason is that the ratio is consistent with several forms of data error, such as age misreporting, which we assume to be zero in the simulations of coverage error.

The ratios in the cumulated series are within 5% of unity up to about age 80. "Within 5% of unity" is an arbitrarily-chosen criterion to gauge the degree to which the calculated ratio deviates from the value where the enumerated population equals the expected population. Beyond age 80, in contrast, the ratios show a rapid increase to levels far above 1.00. (We identify the beginning of a "rapid change" arbitrarily as the point where the ratio's rate of change from the previous age sustains a value greater than or equal to one percent). At the height of the divergence at age 92+, for instance, a ratio value of 1.2428 was found for females, which means that over 24 percent more white females aged 92 and above were enumerated at the time of the second census as were expected based on the number enumerated ten years earlier in the first census in conjunction with intercensal deaths and intercensal migrations. Ratios that are greater than 1.00 are consistent with a Census Bureau conclusion (US Bureau of the Census, 1988; Robinson et al., 1993) that an increase in coverage completeness occurred between 1970 and 1980, which may reflect undercount in the 1970 census, overcount in 1980, or illegal immigration. After age 92+, a clear downward trend is noted for the duration of the cumulated series. Note, however, that the single age series continues its upward trend; the cumulated series is being pulled down by the particularly low centenarian ratio discussed earlier. A s shown in Figure 6.1, the white pattern in 1970-80 is generally above unity and rising with age (up to age 100). As demonstrated in Chapter 5, the pattern of ratios that lie about 1.00 and rise with age is consistent with several forms of data error. The two most plausible patterns of data error are:

1) Net undercount in the 1970 census combined with accurate coverage in the death registration. This speculation is supported for simulations which shows that, when net undercount in the first census is combined with accurate death registration data, the ratio series will decline, regardless of the pattern of coverage error in the second census.

2) Roughly equal probabilities of age overstatement in deaths and in both censuses, a suggestion also supported by simulations.

The former explanation is more likely to be correct. If the pattern of the ratios resulted from similar tendencies for age misstatement in deaths and censuses, one would expect that pattern to continue into the 1980-90 decade, particularly since the 1980 census is involved in both comparisons. And one would not expect cultural predispositions to misstate age to disappear suddenly. But, as will be shown, the 1980-90 pattern of ratios for whites shows remarkable consistency.

A second reason for accepting the first explanation is that the Census Bureau has concluded that the 1970 census is less complete than the 1980 census (US Bureau of the Census, 1988; Robinson, et al., 1993). This conclusion is partially based on demographic analysis and hence is not entirely independent of the kind of evidence under review. However, their demographic analysis is weighted heavily towards ages that are younger than those considered here. Furthermore, the conclusion that census coverage improved is also supported by their post-enumeration program in which individuals in the census are matched against other data systems.

In order to examine the plausibility of our interpretation, we have experimented with different assumed patterns and magnitudes of error in the 1970-1980 white male data sources. Our investigation resulted in a corrected set of estimates in which the pattern of ratios hovers around 1.00 and shows little or no age trend.

In summary, the pattern of ratios that lie above 1.00 and rise with age, as observed for white males and white females in the 1970 to 1980 intercensal period, is consistent with several forms of data error. We believe, however, that the principal cause is the relative incompleteness of the 1970 census relative to the 1980 census and to death registration. Since conventional mortality estimates at older ages are generally calculated by combining numerators from death registration with denominators from population counts, mortality estimates for the US white population which use the 1970 census are likely to overstate mortality.

White Males and Females in 1980-1990 Intercensal Period

Figure 6.2 presents the ratios of observed to expected population for the white male and white female populations in the 1980-1990 intercensal period. In the series that examines the ratios at individual ages, the ratios (in 1990) were invariably within five percent of unity at all single years of age between 50 and 87. In fact, our arbitrarily-chosen criterion to judge the degree of consistency is too lenient at five percent for whites in the 1980-1990 intercensal period. In most single-year ages, the ratio fell within two percent of unity, and often within one percent.

These highly consistent ratios are far better than in most European countries and equivalent to the pattern of ratios found in Sweden and the Netherlands, countries with highly efficient population registers (Condran et al., 1991). The consistency during 1980-1990 is much greater than that in other English-speaking countries: England and Wales, Canada, Australia, and New Zealand.

Figure 6.2

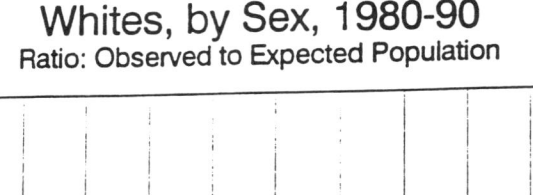

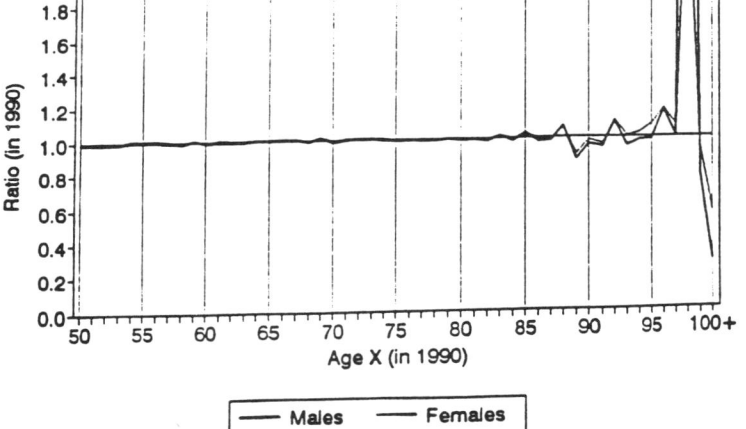

Whites, by Sex, 1980-90
Ratio: Observed to Expected Population

RESULTS FOR AFRICAN AMERICANS

General Discussion of the Declining Ratio Series

In contrast to the differing age pattern of the ratios observed for the white populations between the two intercensal periods, the pattern of ratios for African Americans is far more consistent over time. Figures 6.3 and 6.4 present the results for African Americans in the two intercensal periods: 1970-1980 and 1980-1990.

144   *Racial Differences in Life Expectancy*

Figure 6.3
Blacks, by Sex, 1970-80
Ratio: Observed to Expected Population

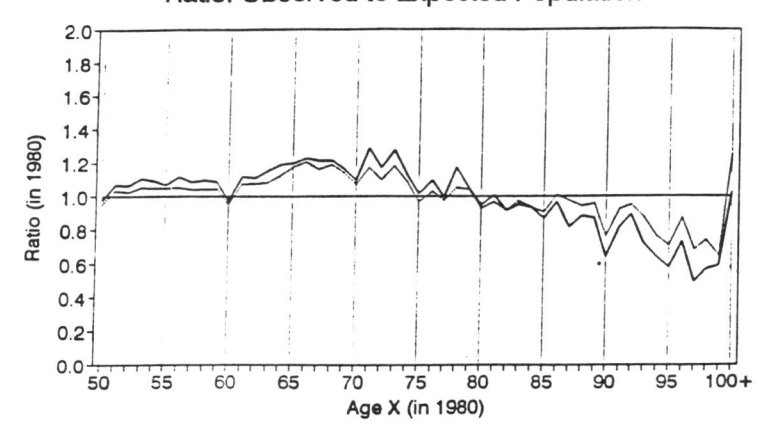

Figure 6.4
Blacks, by Sex, 1980-90
Ratio: Observed to Expected Population

——— Males   ——— Females

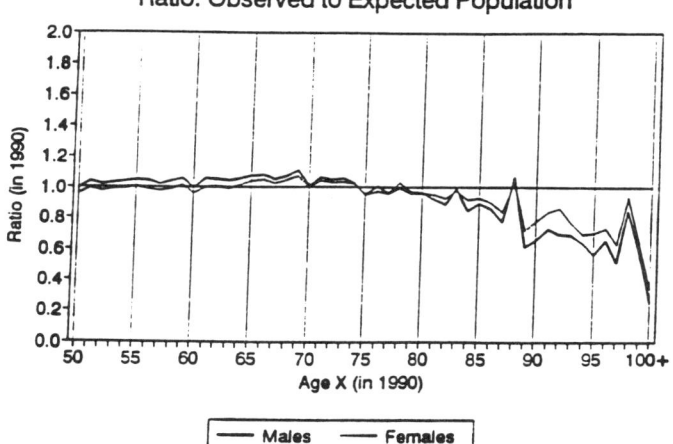

US Errors and their Effects on Life Expectancy

As observed in Figures 6.3 and 6.4, which present the results for blacks in the two intercensal periods, the pattern is characterized by:

1. Ratios that are typically above unity before age 75. For instance, between exact ages 61 and 79 in the 1970-80 period for black males, the actual population in 1980 generally exceeded the expected population by 2 to 29 percent.

2. Ratios begin to fall around age 70 for both sexes in both periods, and continue declining through higher ages (through age 100 in 1970-80).

3. Troughs in the ratios, particularly at ages ending in -0, -5, -7, and -9 are evident.

While the age-pattern is consistent for African Americans of both sexes and across both time periods, it differs markedly from the patterns observed for whites in the same years. The deviation between the actual population enumerated at the time of the second census and the expected population is much larger at the "younger" ages in the series (i.e., at ages less than 65) in the black populations relative to white. Second, the black population experiences a rapid *decrease* in the ratio series in both intercensal periods, while whites experience increases in 1970-1980 and consistent ratios in 1980-1990. Finally, rapid movement away from unity begins at an earlier age in the black series. In the 1970-1980 intercensal period, for instance, white male ratios approximated 1.00 through age 85 while divergence from unity began as early as age 68 for African American males.

The fact that ratios are generally higher for blacks at a particular age in 1970-80 than in 1980-90 is consistent with relative undercount in the 1970 census. As noted earlier, such an undercount is also likely to have occurred among whites. The undercount, however, is insufficient to explain the declining ratio series.

The falling pattern of falling ratios above age 70 for African Americans is consistent with two principal explanations:

1. Deaths are underregistered for the African American population relative to completeness of census coverage.

2. Age overstatement is greater in censuses than in death registration.

Coale and Kisker (1990) lean toward the former explanation. They note that populations reconstructed from deaths, using variable-r procedures (Preston and Coale, 1982), are too small relative to census counts in 1980 above age 65, suggesting relative underregistration of deaths. They also note that fewer African American deaths are recorded at advanced ages in vital registration than in Medicare deaths.

However, both observations are also consistent with ages being overstated in censuses (and Medicare) relative to death registration. That such a pattern exists is strongly supported by a direct match of death certificates in 1960 to records for the same individuals in the 1960 census of population (NCHS, 1968; Hambright, 1969). For either males or females, the total number of deaths above age 50 when deaths are classified according to census age are within 1% of the total number of deaths when classified according to death certificate age. However, at ages 65+, "census age" deaths are 15.4% greater than "death certificate age" deaths for females and 7.1% greater for males. At age 75+, the disparities are 23.3% and 17.8%, respectively, and at age 85+, 39.2% and 17.6%.

These large discrepancies in age reporting between censuses and deaths are capable of accounting for the declining pattern of ratios above age 70 that is demonstrated on Figures 6.3 and 6.4. Elo and Preston (1993) calculate the R_x values for African Americans between 1950-60 and 1960-70, periods that bound the 1960 census-death certificate match. They show that, if ages at death are "corrected" to make them consistent with the age reporting in censuses, the pattern of declining ratios is eliminated.

A final issue evaluates the extent of reporting preference for ages ending in particular digits. We again employed Myers' Blended Method (1940) to analyze black males aged 50 up to age 90 in the 1970 and the 1980 censuses. Referring to Table 6.x, a higher level of age heaping is observed in the black male population than that which was measured for white males. The summary index, which measures the minimum proportion of persons in the population for whom an age with an incorrect final digit is recorded (Shryock and Siegel, 1976), measures only 0.75 for the white males population aged 50 to 89 in 1970, but measured 3.03 for black males of the same ages. The 1980 black population had a lower summary index (2.40) of age heaping, although it remained higher than the comparable white value (0.83). Eight terminal ages (except 2 and 7) had worse heaping in 1970 relative to 1960.

Table 5.8
Calculation of a Preference Index for Terminal Digits by Myers' Blended Method for US Black Males Aged 50-89 in the 1970-1980 Intercensal Period

Terminal Digit X		Blended 1970 Census	Blended 1980 Census	Blended Deaths
0	Percent Distrib.	10.88	10.35	10.41
	Over/Under Expected?	Over	Over	Over
1	Percent Distrib.	9.08	9.42	9.31
	Over/Under Expected?	Under	Under	Under
2	Percent Distrib.	9.60	9.52	9.51
	Over/Under Expected?	Under	Under	Under
3	Percent Distrib.	9.29	9.39	9.63
	Over/Under Expected?	Under	Under	Under
4	Percent Distrib.	10.11	10.06	10.06
	Over/Under Expected?	Over	Over	Over
5	Percent Distrib.	10.49	10.35	10.06
	Over/Under Expected?	Over	Over	Over
6	Percent Distrib.	9.64	9.94	9.78
	Over/Under Expected?	Under	Under	Under
7	Percent Distrib.	10.30	10.47	10.00
	Over/Under Expected?	Over	Over	Exact
8	Percent Distrib.	9.35	9.73	9.93
	Over/Under Expected?	Under	Under	Under
9	Percent Distrib.	11.26	10.75	11.31
	Over/Under Expected?	Over	Over	Over
Summary Index of Prefer.		3.03	2.49	1.84

Source: Adapted from: Myers, R.J. 1940. Errors and bias in the reporting of ages in census data. *Transactions of the Actuarial Society of America*, 41, part 2(104):413.

Notes: (1) "% distribution": proportion of total population reporting on the terminal digit; (2) "summary index of age preference" for all terminal digits: 1/2 the sum of absolute deviations from 10%. If age heaping is nonexistent, index would be zero. The index is an estimate of the minimum proportion of persons in the pop. for whom an age with an incorrect final digit is reported (Shryock and Siegel, 1976).

We also investigated the degree of terminal digit preference in the registered deaths in the 1970-1980 intercensal period. We found lower levels of digit preference in deaths (1.84) relative to the two African American censuses, but more age heaping than observed in the white data sources.

Based on calculations using Myers' Blended Method, the following generalizations can be made about age heaping in the black male population aged 50 to 89 in the 1970 to 1980 intercensal period:

1. Higher levels of digit preference are evident in all three data sources relative to the same sources for whites.

2. Based on the summary index of age heaping, the 1970 census contains the most heaping error, followed by the 1980 census and then death registration.

3. The number of persons reported with terminal digits 1, 2, 3, 6, and 8 was less than that expected in all three sources.

4. The number of persons reported with terminal digits 0, 4, 5, and 9 was more than the expected value in all three sources.

5. The remaining terminal digit -7 was higher than expected in the two censuses and was exact (no deviation between the calculated and the expected value) in deaths.

6. Some differences were observed in the terminal age preferences of whites versus those of African Americans. For instance, the number of whites with terminal age -6 was consistently overstated, while the number of African Americans with the same terminal age was understated.

HOW SENSITIVE ARE OUR RESULTS TO CHOICE OF DATA SOURCES?

A number issues related to data and methodology were identified in the process of completing this thesis, including:

1. Which 1970 data source provides the best approximation of the enumerated 1970 population after correction of the

centenarian problem?

2. Are race-modified or race-unmodified statistics the appropriate data source?

3. What is the effect of exclusion of undocumented aliens in the estimation procedures?

The effect of our choices on the intercensal ratios of observed to expected population was investigated. The general conclusion is that the ratios were highly robust to the specified issues.

Comparison of the Effects of Two Different Sources of 1970 Census Data on the Ratios in 1980

We discussed problems in the official count of the 1970 census in earlier chapters. Inaccuracies included: (1) a conspicuous overcount of the centenarian population, likely the result of misunderstanding of the Census questionnaire; (2) misclassification of the population by race; and, (3) errors in the counts of local areas.

Two sets of 1970 data which adjust for one or more of the inaccuracies were discussed. The first, tabulations by Shrestha, adjust for the large centenarian overcount by utilizing Medicare estimates of the 1970 population aged 100 and over and distributing the "excess" centenarians pro rata. The second, unpublished tabulations from the Census Bureau, adjust for all three problems.

We utilize the Census Bureau tabulations. Their use was favored because adjustments were made for all three problems although it was recognized that the procedures used to estimate the size of the centenarian population were flawed.

In order to ascertain the sensitivity of the ratios of observed to expected population in 1980 to the choice of 1970 census estimate, we compare ratios obtained in each instance. While the estimated counts of the centenarian population differ significantly between the two sources, the intercensal ratios are nearly identical. Because the population aged 100 and over in 1980 is estimated by the forward survival of the population aged *90 and over* in 1970, the differences in the centenarian estimates are diluted by the absolute size of the population aged 90+ in 1970.

Sensitivity of Ratio Results to the Use of Race-Modified Census Tabulation in the Estimation Procedure

In earlier chapters, we discussed race misclassification in the official decennial censuses. The principal problem was that a large number (6.8 million in 1980 and 9.2 million in 1990) of Spanish-origin persons chose to write-in a response to the race question rather than choose one of the designated categories. Since only the censuses have this "not specified" race category, comparison of Census results to other data sources (such as vital registration and Medicare) may cause biases. In Chapter 3, we provided justification for use of the modified race tabulations. In order to judge the sensitivity of the intercensal ratios of observed to expected population, we compared results which include the race modifications to the official statistics (which exclude the modifications).

In both the race-modified and race-unmodified tabulations in the 1970-1980 intercensal period, the baseline population is unpublished Census estimates for 1970 received from the US Bureau of the Census. The unmodified 1980 census refers to the official count (US Bureau of the Census, 1983a). The 6.8 million persons identified as "not specified" race in the official tabulations have been transferred to specific races in the modified 1980 statistics (US Bureau of the Census, 1983b). As observed in Figures 5.J.a, the ratios of observed to expected population in 1980 for both white males and black males are highly robust to the choice of official or race-modified 1980 tabulations.

For the 1980-1990 intercensal period, official tabulations (US Bureau of the Census, 1983a, 1991) of the population were utilized for the unmodified calculations. Race-modified tabulations were utilized for both the 1980 and 1990 censuses. As noted earlier, to construct the 1980 modified series, the US Bureau of the Census transferred 6.8 million individuals from "non-specified" to designated racial categories. In 1990, the transfer involved 9.2 million. The 1990 modification also included an age modification.

While the pattern of the ratios of observed to expected population in 1990 remain similar whether unmodified or race-modified statistics are utilized, the ratios are smoother with use of the modified statistics. More spikes in the series are observed with use of the unmodified statistics.

Sensitivity of Ratio Results to the Exclusion of Illegal Aliens from the Estimation Procedure

We noted that undocumented residents are excluded in our constructed immigration series. We argued that exclusion of this group is justified on two accounts. First, in the old-age categories, even the most exaggerated estimates of the number of illegal aliens are small relative to the number of deaths as a source of change in the composition of the cohorts. Second, estimates of the magnitude and the characteristic distribution of the illegal population vary widely due to insufficient data collection instruments in the United States.

In order to judge the sensitivity of the intercensal ratios of observed/expected population, we compared results which exclude estimates of the undocumented population to results which include estimates of their size. We use utilize estimates from the US Bureau of the Census which are classified by age, race, and sex.

The results are highly robust to the inclusion (or exclusion) of the undocumented residents. The pattern remained identical. The magnitudes of the ratios did deviate between the two sources, but the differences were of only thousandth's of a point at a given age. In fact, the differences between the two sets of estimates generally were less than .003, with the exception of whites at the very extreme ages (96 and over). The ratios which exclude illegal aliens surpass the values which exclude them. A net inflow of illegal aliens causes an inflation in the denominator of the R_x equation which results in a decrease in the ratio values.

If the Census Bureau estimates of the illegal population are reasonable approximations, the sensitivity analysis demonstrated that the exclusion of the illegal aliens from intercensal estimation of ratios of observed/expected population does not bias the results. Furthermore, the analysis illustrates that substantial movements of undocumented immigrants are required to effect only changes in the values of the ratio series.

CONCLUSION

In this chapter, the intercensal cohort method of data evaluation was employed to evaluate the quality of old age mortality data in the United States. Such estimation was done for each sex and by race (black, white) for two intercensal periods: 1970-1980 and

1980-1990. Analysis of the ratios of observed to expected population at the time of the second census indicates that, at the older ages:

1. The degree of inconsistency increases with age in all four sex-race combinations;

2. The inconsistencies in the ratios are worse for blacks than for whites;

3. Within race, the ratios of observed to expected population calculated for males showed remarkably similar patterns of change to those of females;

4. Big improvement in the consistency of the ratios is observed for whites between the 1970-80 and 1980-90 intercensal periods.

5. Different patterns of error affect the white and black populations.

Specifically, white data for the 1980-90 decade were found to be remarkably consistent. Data quality up to age 95 approaches that of Sweden and the Netherlands, countries that maintain highly efficient population registers. Less consistency was observed for whites during the 1970-80 intercensal period. We provide evidence that the principal explanation for the pattern of inconsistencies is the combination of net undercount in the 1970 census with overcount in the 1980 census and accurate death statistics.

African American data are far less consistent. Above age 70, the enumerated population falls increasingly below the expected population in both 1980 and 1990. It appears likely that the major reason for this pattern is that ages are more overstated in censuses relative to death registration. This inconsistency was revealed in a 1960 match of death certificates and census records, and it appears to have continued to the present. Furthermore, correction of the initial data sources for the assumed pattern of error greatly improves the ratio series of observed to expected population.

Reasons why African American ages are overstated in censuses relative to deaths are not obvious. The pattern does not appear until the 1940 census, the first census after Social Security legislation was passed. At that census, a large surplus of African American persons aged 65-69 and 70-74 appears, and a deficit of persons aged 50-64 (Elo and Preston, 1993). This surplus also appears, although in increasingly attenuated form, in subsequent censuses. Whatever its source, we believe that the principal explanation of the large inconsistencies between the censuses and death registration for the African American population is a pattern of age overstatement in censuses relative to death registration. Such a pattern implies that recorded death rates above age 65 for African-Americans are likely to be seriously underestimated. A crossover between black and white death rates may indeed occur at advanced ages, but basing such a conclusion on census and vital registration data is risky. These data are simply too inconsistent with one another to allow death rates at advanced ages to be estimated with any confidence. This result is also consistent with work by Elo and Preston (1994), who evaluated the quality of vital statistics and census data for estimating African-American mortality over a period of six decades. They used demographic techniques to demonstrate that coventionally constructed African-American death rates may be seriously flawed as early as age 50. Their results suggest that,if a racial crossover in death rates occurs, the age pattern of mortality among African Americans must be far outside the range observed in population with more accurate data.

Bibliography

Bean, F.D., A.G. King and J.S. Passel. 1983. The number of illegal migrants of Mexican origin in the United States: sex ratio-based estimates for 1980. *Demography*, 20:99-109.

Bennett, N.G. and S. Horiuchi. 1981. Estimating the completeness of death registration in a closed population. *Population Index*, 47(2):207-221.

_____. 1984. Mortality estimation from registered deaths in less developed countries. *Demography*, 21(2):217-233.

Butz, W.P. 1991. Evaluation of the 1990 census. Paper presented at the annual meeting of the Population Association of America, Washington, D.C.

CENIET (1981). Informe Final: Los Trabajadores Mexicanos en los Estados Unidos (Encuesta Nacional de Emigracion a la Frontera Norte del Pais y a los Estados Unidos--ENEFNEU--). Secretaria del Trabajo y Prevision Social. Centro Nacional de Informacion y Estadisticas del Trabajo. Mexico City.

Coale, A.J. and E.E. Kisker. 1986. Mortality crossovers: reality or bad data? *Population Studies*, 40(3):389-401.

Coale, A.J. and E.E. Kisker. 1990. Defects in data on old-age mortality in the United States: new procedures for calculating mortality schedules and life tables at the highest ages. *Asian and Pacific Population Forum*, 4(1):1-31.

Coale, A.J. and N.W. Rives, Jr. 1973. A statistical reconstruction of the black population of the United States, 1880-1970: Estimates of true numbers by age and sex, birth rates, and total fertility. *Population Index*, 39(1):3-36.

Coale, A.J. and M. Zelnik. 1963. *New Estimates of Fertility and Population in the United States*. Princeton, NJ: Princeton University Press.

Condran, G.A., C.L. Himes, and S.H. Preston. 1991. Old-age mortality patterns in low-mortality countries: an evaluation of population and death data at advanced ages, 1950 to present. *Population Bulletin of the United Nations*, no. 30:23-60.

Elo, I.T. and S.H. Preston. 1991. Effects of early-life conditions on adult mortality: a review. *Population Index*, 58(2):186-212.

Elo, I.T. and S.H. Preston. 1994. Estimating African-American mortality from inaccurate data. *Demography*, 31(3):427-458.

Elo, I.T. and S.H. Preston. 1993. New estimates of old-age mortality among African Americans, 1930-1990. Paper presented at the Population Association of America meetings, Cincinnati.

Ewbank, D.C. 1981. *Age Misreporting and Age Selective Underenumeration: Sources, Patterns, and Consequences for Demographic Analysis*. National Academy of Sciences, Committee on Population and Demography. Report No. 4. Washington, D.C.: National Academy Press.

Farley, R. and W.R. Allen. 1987. *The Color Line and the Quality of Life in America*. New York: Russell Sage.

Farley, D.O., T. Richards, and R.M. Bell. No Date. How good are estimates of infant mortality rates? A draft of a paper produced at RAND Corporation.

Garcia y Griego, M., 1980. *El volumen de la Migracion de Mexicanos no Documentados a los Estados Unidos (Nuevas Hipotesis)*. Secretaria del Trabajo y Prevision Social. Centro Nacional de Informacion y Estadisticas del Trabajo. Mexico City.

Goldberg, H. 1974. Estimates of emigration from Mexico and illegal entry into the United States, 1960-1970, by the residual method. Unpublished graduate research paper. Center for Population Research. Georgetown University, Washington, D.C.

Hambright, T.Z. 1969. Comparison of information on death certificates and matching 1960 census records: age, marital status, nativity, and country of origin. *Demography*, 6(4).

Heer, D.M. 1979. What is the annual net flow of undocumented Mexican immigrants to the United States? *Demography*, 16(3):417-423.

Hill, K. 1985. Illegal aliens: an assessment. In: Panel on Immigration Statistics. *Immigration Statistics, A Story of Neglect*. Washington, DC: National Academy Press.

Himes, C.L. and C. Clogg. 1992. An overview of "demographic analysis" as a method for evaluation census coverage in the United States. Forthcoming in *Population Index*, Draft dated October 8, 1992.

Hollmann, F.W. and G. Spencer. 1992a. Discontinuities in age and race data from the 1990 census. Paper presented at the annual meeting of the Population Association of America, Denver, Co.

_____. 1992b. Verbal presentation and personal communication. Population Association of America meetings, Denver, Colorado.

Horiuchi, S. and S.H. Preston. 1988. Age-specific growth rates: the legacy of past population dynamics. *Demography*, 25(3):429-441.

Horn, M.C. 1985. A cohort analysis of sex differentials in mortality among older adults: England and Wales. Unpublished doctoral dissertation. University of Pennsylvania, Graduate Group in Demography.

Kermack, W.O., A.G. McKendrick and P.L. McKinlay. 1934a. Death rates in Great Britain and Sweden: some regularities and their significance. *The Lancet*, 1:698-703.

Kermack, W.O., A.G. McKendrick and P.L. McKinlay. 1934b. Death rates in Great Britain and Sweden: expression of specific mortality rates as products of two factors, and some consequences thereof. *Journal of Hygiene*, 34:433-457.

Kestenbaum, B. 1992. A description of the extreme aged population based on improved Medicare enrollment data. *Demography*, 29(4):565-580.

Kestenbaum, B. 1990. A matched-records study of age at death information. Paper presented at the annual meeting of the American Statistical Association, Anaheim, Ca.

Kestenbaum, Bert, NO DATE. A description of the extreme aged population based on improved Medicare enrollment data. [Draft based on earlier versions of papers presented at Population Association of America, Baltimore, 1989 and American Statistical Association, Anaheim, 1990].

Kitagawa, E.M. and P.M. Hauser. 1973. *Differential Mortality in the United States: a Study of Socioeconomic Epidemiology.* Cambridge, Massachusetts: Harvard University Press.

Lancaster, C. and F.J. Scheuren. 1978. Counting the uncountable illegals: some initial statistical speculations employing capture-recapture techniques. 1977 Proceedings of the Social Statistics Section. Part 1, pp. 530-535. American Statistical Association.

Manton, K.G. 1980. Sex and race specific mortality differentials in multiple cause of death data. *The Gerontologist*, 20(4).

-----. 1982. Differential life expectancy: possible explanations during the later ages. In: R.C. Manuel (ed.). *Minority Aging: Sociological and Social Psychological Issues.* Westport, Connecticut/London, England: Greenwood Press: pp. 63-68.

Manton, K.G. and S.S. Poss. 1977. The black/white mortality crossover: possible racial differences in the intrinsic rate of aging. *Black Aging*, Vol. 3.

Manton, K.G., S.S. Poss, and S. Wing. 1979. The black-white mortality crossover: investigation from the perspective of the components of aging. *The Gerontologist*, 19(3):291-300.

Manton, K.G. and E. Stallard. 1981. Methods for evaluating the heterogeneity of human populations using vital statistics data: explaining the black/white mortality crossover by a model of mortality selection. *Human Biology*, 53(1):47-67.

Manton, K.G., E. Stallard, and J.W. Vaupel. 1986. Alternative models for the heterogeneity of mortality risks among the aged. *Journal of the American Statistical Association*, 81:635-644.

Markides, K.S. and C.H. Mindel. 1987. *Aging and Ethnicity*. Newbury Park, CA: Sage Publications: Sage Library of Social Research #163.

McCord, C. and H.P. Freeman. 1990. Excess mortality in Harlem. *New England Journal of Medicine*, 322:172-177.

McKinney, N.R., E.W. Fernandez, and W.T. Masumura. 1980. The quality of race and Spanish-origin information reported in the 1980 census. Proceedings of the Social Statistics Section of the American Statistical Association.

Murray, C.B., S. Khatib, and M. Jackson. 1989. Social indices and the black elderly: a comparative life cycle approach to the study of double jeopardy. In: R.L. Jones (ed.), *Black Adult Development and Aging*. Berkeley, CA: Cobb and Henry Publishers. pp. 167-185.

Myers, R.J. 1940. Errors and bias in the reporting of ages in census data. *Transactions of the Actuarial Society of America*, 41. Pt. 2 (104):411-415.

Nam, C.B. and K.A. Ockay. 1978. Causes of death which contribute to the mortality crossover effect. *Social Biology*, 25:306-314.

National Center for Health Statistics. 1968. *Comparability of age on the death certificate and matching census record: United States- May - August 1960*; Vital and Health Statistics: Data Evaluation and Methods Research. By Thea Zelman Hambright. Series 2, No. 29.

_____. 1970-1988. *Mortality Detail Files* (and codebooks). Data were made available by the Inter-University Consortium for Political and Social Research, University of Michigan.

_____. 1975. US Decennial Life Tables: 1969-71. Vol. 1, No. 1. Rockville, Maryland: US Department of Health, Education, and Welfare.

_____. 1985. US Decennial Life Tables: 1979-81. Vol. 1, No 1. DHHS Publication No. (PHS)85-1150-1

_____. 1989. Births, marriages, divorces, and deaths for January-December 1989. *Monthly* vital statistics report. Vol. 38, nos. 1-12. Hyattsville, Maryland: Public Health Service.

_____. 1990. Births, marriages, divorces, and deaths for January-March 1990. *Monthly* vital statistics report. Vol. 39, nos. 1-3. Hyattsville, Maryland: Public Health Service.

_____. 1992. Advanced report on final mortality statistics, 1989. Monthly vital statistics report. Vol. 40, no. 8, supp. 2. Hyattsville, Maryland: Public Health Service.

National Office of Vital Statistics. 1950. *Births and birth rates in the entire United States, 1909 to 1948*, Vital Statistics -Special Reports, By P.K. Whelpton. 33(8). Washington, DC.

Panel on Immigration Statistics, 1985. *Immigration Statistics, A Story of Neglect*. Washington, DC: National Academy Press.

Passel, J.S. and P.A. Berman. 1986. Quality of 1980 census data for American Indians. *Social Biology*, Vol. 33:163-182.

Passel, J.S. and J.G. Robinson. 1988. Methodology for developing estimates of coverage in the 1980 census based on demographic analysis: immigration statistics (legal). US Bureau of the Census, Preliminary Evaluation Results Memorandum No. 113. Draft dated September 1988.

Poe, G.S., E. Powell-Griner, J.K. Mc Laughlin, P.J. Placek, G.B. Thompsen, and K. Robinson. 1992. Comparability of reporting of demographic items between the death certificate and the 1986 National Mortality Followback Survey. National Center for Health Statistics: Data Evaluation and Methods Research: Series 2. Draft dated 5/14/1992.

Pressat, R. 1988. *The Dictionary of Demography*. Edited by Christopher Wilson. Oxford/New York: Basil Blackwell Ltd, Blackwell Reference.

Preston, S.H. 1993. Demographic change in the United States, 1970-2050. Forthcoming in Sylvester Scheiber, ed. *Demography and Retirement: The 21st Century*. New York: Praeger Press.

Preston, S.H. (Principle Investigator), I. Rosenwaike, I. Elo, A. McDaniel, and H. Smith. 1991. African-American Mortality: 1930-1990. A grant application submitted to the Department of Health and Human Services, unpublished.

Preston, S.H. and N.G. Bennett. 1983. A census-based method for estimating adult mortality. *Population Studies*, 37:91-104.

Preston, S.H. and A.J. Coale. 1982. Age structure, growth, attrition, and accession: a new synthesis. *Population Index*, 48(2):217-259.

Preston, S.H. and E. van de Walle. 1978. Urban French mortality in the nineteenth century. *Population Studies*, 32:275-297.

Rives, N.W. 1977. The effect of census errors on life table estimates of black mortality. *Public Health Briefs*, 67:867-868.

Robinson, J.G. 1980. Estimating the approximate size of the illegal alien population in the United States by the comparative trend analysis of age-specific death rates. *Demography*, 17(2):159-176.

_____. 1992. Personal communication.

Robinson, J.G., B. Ahmed, P. Das Gupta, K.A. Woodrow. 1992. Estimation of population coverage in the 1990 United States census based on demographic analysis. Forthcoming in: Journal of the American Statistical Association, Special Section on the 1990 Undercount. Draft dated 8/20/92.

Robinson, J.G, P.D. Gupta and B. Ahmed. 1990. A case study in the investigation of errors in estimates of coverage based on demographic analysis: black adults aged 35 to 54 in 1980. Paper presented at the annual meeting of American Statistical Association, Anaheim, CA.

Robinson, J.G. and S. Lapham. 1991. Inconsistencies in race classifications of the demographic estimates and the census. 1990 Decennial Census, Preliminary Research and Evaluation Memorandum (PREM) No. 82, Demographic Analysis Evaluation Project D9.

Robinson, J.G., D.L. Word and G. Spencer. 1991. Uncertainty for models to translate 1990 census concepts into historical racial classifications. 1990 Decennial Census, Preliminary Research and Evaluation Memorandum (PREM) No. 81, Demographic Analysis Evaluation Project D8.

Rosenwaike, I. and B. Logue. 1983. Accuracy of death certificate ages for the extreme aged. *Demography*, 20(4):569-585.

Shryock, H.S. and J.S. Siegel. 1976. *The Methods and Material of Demography*. Orlando, Florida: Academic Press, Inc. (Harcourt Brace Jovanovich, Publishers): Studies in Population Series.

Siegel, J.S. 1974. Estimates of coverage of the population by sex, race, and age in the 1970 census. *Demography*, 11(1):1-23.

Siegel, J.S. and M. Davidson. 1984. Demographic and socioeconomic aspects of aging in the United States. *Current Population Reports*. Series P-23, no. 138. Bureau of the Census. Washington: US Government Printing Office.

Siegel, J.S. and J.S. Passel. 1976. New estimates of the number of centenarians in the United States. *Journal of the American Statistical Association*, 71(355):559-566.

Sorlie, P.D., E. Rogot, and N.J. Johnson. 1992. Validity of demographic characteristics on the death certificate. *Epidemiology*, 3(2):181-184.

Sprague, T.B. 1800-81. Explanation of a new formula for interpolation. *Journal of the Institute of Actuaries*, 22:270. (Cited in Shyrock and Siegel, 1976, p. 534).

United Nations. 1983. *Manual X: Indirect Techniques for Demographic Estimation*. Population Studies, No. 81. By K. Hill, H. Zlotnik, and J. Trussell. New York: United Nations.

US Bureau of the Census. 1921. *United States Life Tables, 1890, 1901, 1910, and 1901-10*, by James W. Glover, pp. 344-348. (Cited in Shyrock and Siegel, 1976, p. 534).

_____. 1960. *Historical Statistics of the United States: Colonial Times to 1957*. A Statistical Abstract Supplement. Series A.22-23. Washington, D.C.: US Government Printing Office.

_____. 1971. US Census of Population and Housing: 1970. *Data Collection Forms and Procedures*. PHC(R)-2. Washington, D.C.: US Government Printing Office.

_____. 1972a. *General Population Characteristics*, 1970 Census of Population and Housing, Final Report PC(1)-B1, United States Summary, Washington, DC: US Government Printing Office.

_____. 1972b. *General Social and Economic Characteristics*, 1970 Census of Population and Housing, Final Report PC(1)-C1, United States Summary, Washington, DC: US Government Printing Office.

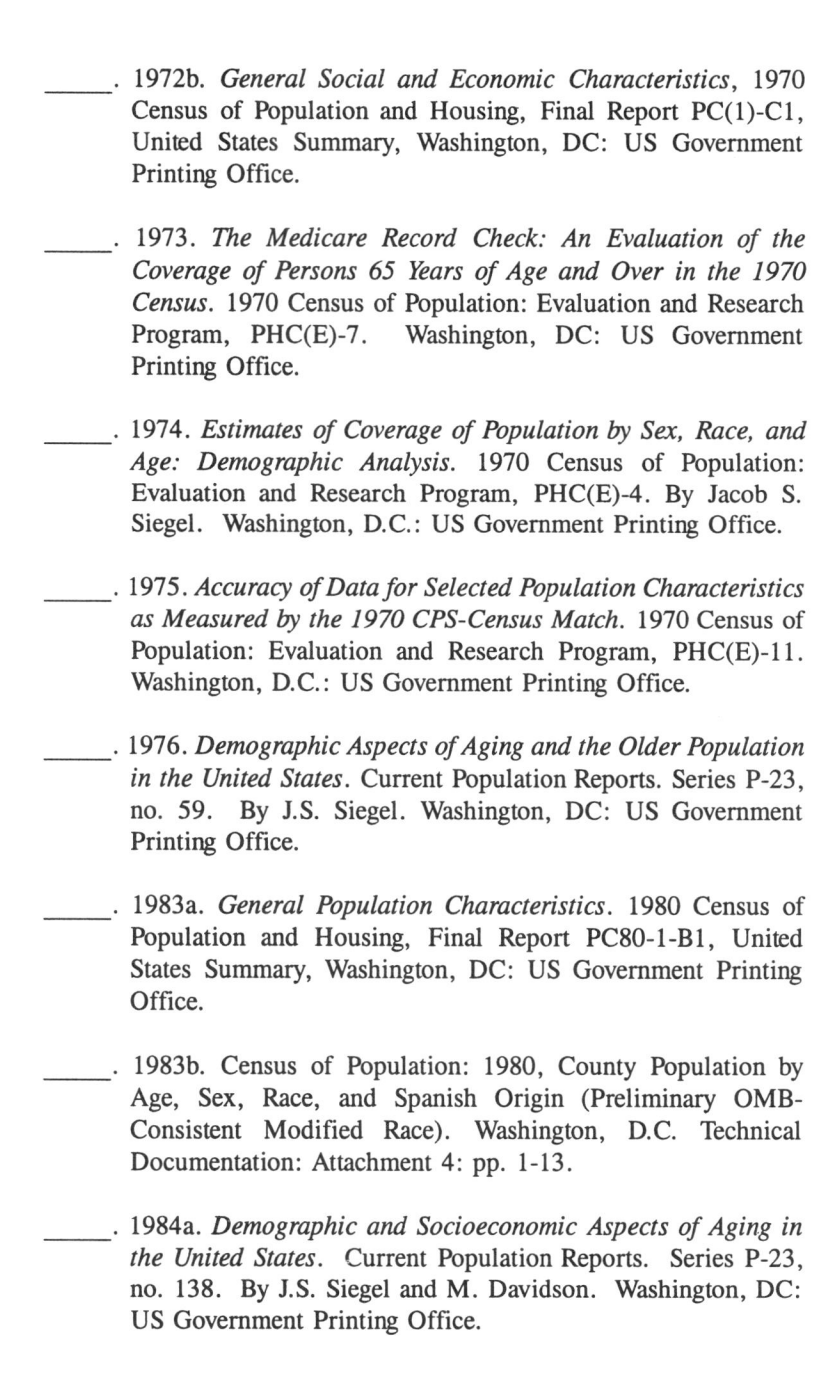

_____. 1973. *The Medicare Record Check: An Evaluation of the Coverage of Persons 65 Years of Age and Over in the 1970 Census*. 1970 Census of Population: Evaluation and Research Program, PHC(E)-7. Washington, DC: US Government Printing Office.

_____. 1974. *Estimates of Coverage of Population by Sex, Race, and Age: Demographic Analysis*. 1970 Census of Population: Evaluation and Research Program, PHC(E)-4. By Jacob S. Siegel. Washington, D.C.: US Government Printing Office.

_____. 1975. *Accuracy of Data for Selected Population Characteristics as Measured by the 1970 CPS-Census Match*. 1970 Census of Population: Evaluation and Research Program, PHC(E)-11. Washington, D.C.: US Government Printing Office.

_____. 1976. *Demographic Aspects of Aging and the Older Population in the United States*. Current Population Reports. Series P-23, no. 59. By J.S. Siegel. Washington, DC: US Government Printing Office.

_____. 1983a. *General Population Characteristics*. 1980 Census of Population and Housing, Final Report PC80-1-B1, United States Summary, Washington, DC: US Government Printing Office.

_____. 1983b. Census of Population: 1980, County Population by Age, Sex, Race, and Spanish Origin (Preliminary OMB-Consistent Modified Race). Washington, D.C. Technical Documentation: Attachment 4: pp. 1-13.

_____. 1984a. *Demographic and Socioeconomic Aspects of Aging in the United States*. Current Population Reports. Series P-23, no. 138. By J.S. Siegel and M. Davidson. Washington, DC: US Government Printing Office.

_____. 1984b. Census of Population: 1980. Race detail file. 100% count. Table IV: modified counts (OMB-consistent) by age, race, and sex. Unpublished tabulations.

_____. 1987a. *Estimates of the Population of the United States, by Age, Sex, and Race: 1980 to 1986.* Current Population Reports. Series P-25, no. 1000. Washington, DC: US Government Printing Office.

_____. 1987b. *America's Centenarians: Data from the 1980 Census.* Current Population Reports. Series P-23, no. 153. Washington, DC: US Government Printing Office.

_____. 1987c. *Statistical Abstract of the United States: 1988.* (108th edition). Washington, D.C.: US Government Printing Office.

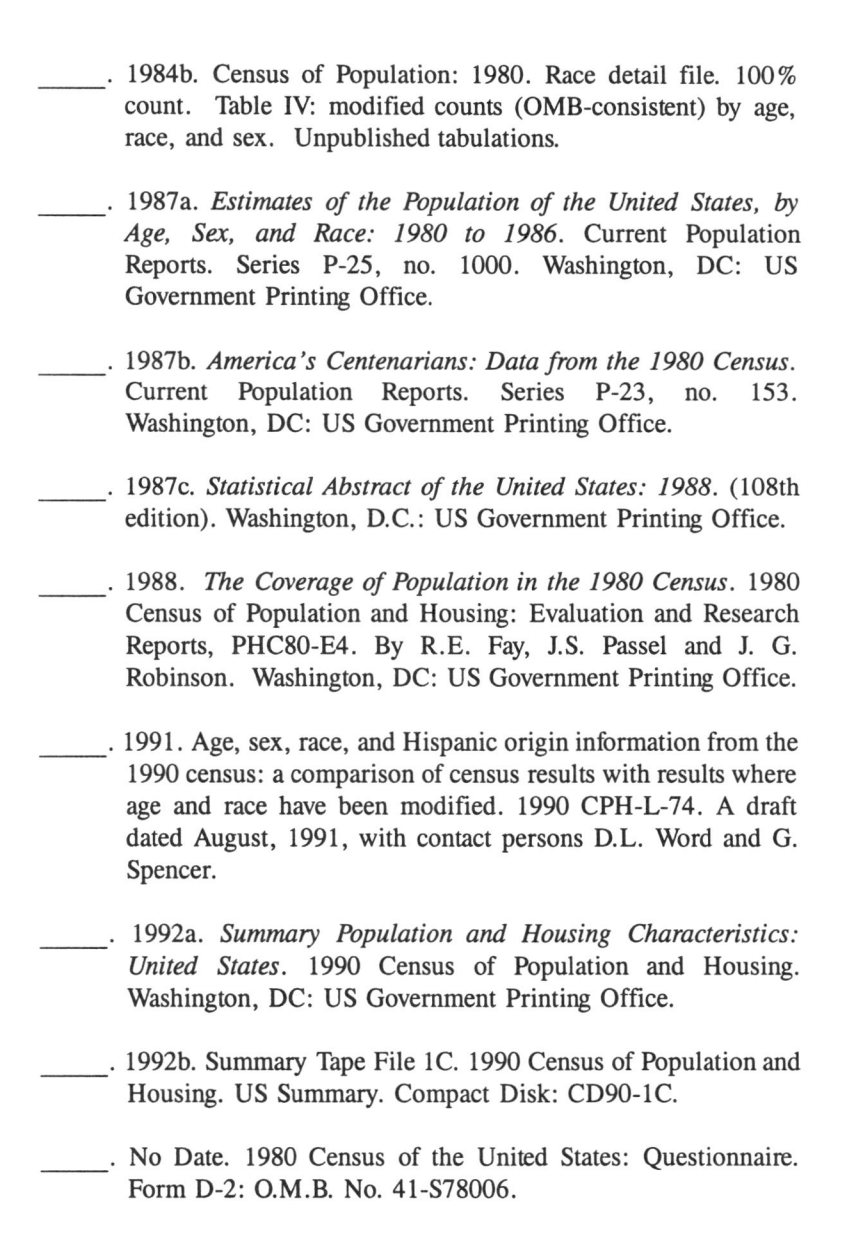

_____. 1988. *The Coverage of Population in the 1980 Census.* 1980 Census of Population and Housing: Evaluation and Research Reports, PHC80-E4. By R.E. Fay, J.S. Passel and J. G. Robinson. Washington, DC: US Government Printing Office.

_____. 1991. Age, sex, race, and Hispanic origin information from the 1990 census: a comparison of census results with results where age and race have been modified. 1990 CPH-L-74. A draft dated August, 1991, with contact persons D.L. Word and G. Spencer.

_____. 1992a. *Summary Population and Housing Characteristics: United States.* 1990 Census of Population and Housing. Washington, DC: US Government Printing Office.

_____. 1992b. Summary Tape File 1C. 1990 Census of Population and Housing. US Summary. Compact Disk: CD90-1C.

_____. No Date. 1980 Census of the United States: Questionnaire. Form D-2: O.M.B. No. 41-S78006.

Warren, R. and J.S. Passel. 1983. Estimates of illegal aliens from Mexico counted in the 1980 United States census. Paper presented at the annual meeting of the Population Association of America, Pittsburgh.

Wilkin, J.C. 1981. Recent trends in the mortality of the aged. *Transactions of the Society of Actuaries*, Vol. XXXIII.

Wing, S., K.G. Manton, E. Stallard, C.G. Hames, and H.A. Tryoler. 1985. The black/white mortality crossover: investigation in a community-based study. *Journal of Gerontology*, 40(1).

Word, D.L. 1993. Personal communication at the Population Association of America meetings, Cincinnati.

Word, D.L. and G. Spencer. 1991. Age, sex, race, and Hispanic-origin information from the 1990 census: a comparison of census results with results where age and race have been modified. 1990 Census: CPH-L-74. Draft dated August, 1991.

Young, C. M. 1978. Cohort analysis of mortality: an historical survey of the literature. Australian National University, Department of Demography: Working Papers in Demography #10: 1-37.

Zelnik, M. 1969. Age patterns of mortality of American Negroes: 1900-02 to 1959-61. *Journal of the American Statistical Association*, 64:433-451.

Author Index

Ahmed, B., 51
Allen, W.R., 9
Bean, F.D., 72
Bell, R.M., 55
Bennett, N.G., 112-114
Berman, P.A., 54
Butz, W. P., 45
CENIET, 64, 72
Clogg, C., 51
Coale, A.J., 4, 6, 8-10, 23, 26, 34, 41, 55, 57, 63-64, 74, 81, 144
Condran, G. A., 4
Elo, I.T., 6, 9, 57-60, 70
Ewbank, D. C., 4
Farley, D.O., 9
Farley, R., 55
Fernandez, E.W., 54
Freeman, H.P., 6, 9
Garcia y Griego, M., 72
Goldberg, H., 72
Gupta, P.D., 51
Hambright, T.Z., 63
Hames, C.G., 10
Hauser, P.M., 10
Heer, D.M., 72
Hill, K., 72
Himes, C.L., 4, 51
Hollmann, F.W., 17-18, 49, 90, 92, 94
Horiuchi, S., 112
Horn, M.C., 9
Jackson, M., 10

Johnson, N.J., 61
Kermack, W.O., 9
Kestenbaum, B., 10, 61-63, 74
Khatib, S., 10
King, A.G., 72
Kisker, E.E., 4, 6, 8-10, 34, 57, 63-64, 74, 81, 144
Kitagawa, E.M., 10
Lancaster, C., 72
Lapham, S., 18, 20, 54-55
Logue, B., 4, 65, 67, 70
Manton, K., 9-10
Markides, K.S., 10
Masumura, W.T., 54
McCord, C., 6, 9
McDaniel, A., 6, 57-60, 70
McKendrick, A.G., 9
McKinney, N.R., 54
McKinlay, P.L., 9
McLaughlin, J.K., 55, 58-60
Mindel, C.H., 10
Murray, C.B., 10
Nam, C. B., 10
National Center for Health Statistics, 8, 57, 63, 74, 95, 97
National Office of Vital Statistics, 41
Ockay, K.A., 10
Panel on Immigration Statistics, 70-71

Passel, J.S., 6, 20-21, 34, 53-54, 71-72, 76, 78, 80-81
Placek, P.J., 55, 58-60
Poe, G.S., 55, 58-60
Poss, S.S., 9
Powell-Griner, E., 55, 58-60
Pressat, R., 4, 53
Preston, S.H., 4, 6, 9-10, 57-60, 64, 70, 112-114, 144
Richards, T., 55
Rives, N.W., 10, 23, 26, 41, 55
Robinson, J.G., 18, 20, 49-51, 53-55, 71, 78, 80, 85, 90
Robinson, K., 55, 58-60
Rogot, E., 61
Rosenwaike, I., 4, 6, 57-60, 65, 67, 70
Schenker, 48, 50
Scheuren, F.J., 72
Shryock, H.S., 3, 102-103

Siegel, J.S., 3, 6, 20-21, 24, 26, 34, 76-78, 80-81, 102-103
Smith, H., 6, 57-60, 70
Sorlie, P.D., 61
Spencer, G., 7, 17-18, 49, 85, 90, 92, 94
Sprague, T.B., 103
Stallard, E., 9-10
Thompsen, G.B., 55, 58-60
Tryoler, H.A., 10
United Nations, 114
Vaupel, J.W., 9
Warren, R., 72
Whelpton, 41
Wilkin, J.C., 72
Wing, S., 9-10
Woodrow-Lafield, K.A., 14, 51
Word, D.L., 7, 85, 90
Young, C.M., 9
Zelnik, M., 6, 10, 23

Content Index

Adult mortality, 9
Age heaping, 13,53-54
Age misreporting, 3, 18, 73, 105-130
Age misreporting:
 patterns of, 128-129
Age overstatement, 4, 107-111
Allocation, 14-18
American Samoa, 14
Armed forces, 13
Asian Indian population, 39
Britain, 9
Census: 1900, 65-70
Census matching study, 4
Centenarian population, 6-8, 20-21, 40
Chicago mortality study, 63
Coding, 3
Content, 18, 21
Correlation bias, 20
Coverage, 13, 18, 21, 73-74, 105-130
Coverage, patterns of, 131
Current Mortality Sample, 74
Current Population Survey, (CPS), 20-21,61,73
Data processing, 3,6
Data sources:
 adjustment of, 73-104
Death registration, 10,57-70
Demographic analysis, 19, 22-27, 41-44, 48, 50-52, 73

Demographic characteristics, 20
Dependency ratio, 5
Diplomats, 13-14
Disease, 9
Early life conditions, 9
Economic deprivation, 9
Enumeration, 13
Evaluation:
 1970 census, 20-38
 1980 census, 39-48
 1990 census, 48-53
 Deaths, 57-70
 Immigration, 70-72
Foreign residents, 13-14
Forward survival, 21
Genetics, 9
Guam, 14
Heterogeneity, 8
Hispanic population, 39,49
Immigration, 70-72, 97-103
Index of inconsistency, 31
Institutionalized population, 13
Intercensal cohort method, 10, 105-107
Intrinsic rate of aging, 8
Life expectancy, 8, 152-153
Life tables, 8
Linkage studies, mortality, 58-63
Massachusetts, 61
Medical intervention, 5

Medicare, 20-21, 27-35, 48, 61, 73
Mortality, 4, 8-10, 57
Mortality crossover, 6, 8-10, 152-153
Myers' summary index, 54, 138-139, 147-148
National Death Index, 61
National Longitudinal Mortality Study, 61
National Mortality Followback Survey, 58-61, 74
Natural selection, 6,8
National Center for Health Statistics, 8,57
Net difference rate, 31
Netherlands, 6-8
New Jersey, 4, 65-70
Nutritional status, 9
Omissions, 38
Pennsylvania, 4, 65-70
PEP/PES, 44-47, 52-53
Population reconstruction, 21
Post enumeration program, 44-48, 52-53
Puerto Rico, 14

Race, 15
Race misreporting/misclassification, 18, 21, 39, 49, 54-55
Racism, 9
Random variability, 20
Record check/linkage, 4, 20, 44-48
Resident population, 14
Results, 131-154
 for whites, 136-143
 for African Americans, 143-148
Sampling error, 20
Selectivity bias, 20
Sensitivity of results, 148-151
Sex, 15
Simulations, 105-130
Social security, 61-70
Survival of the fittest, 8
Sweden, 6-9
Texas, 61
"True" populations:
 derivation of, 111-120
Tuberculosis, 9
Undocumented population, 14